Manual Therapy Approaches in

NEUROPHYSIOTHERAPY

Manual Therapy Approaches in
NEUROPHYSIOTHERAPY

Suvarna Ganvir
BPhT MPhT PGDR FNR CMCL-FAIMER
Fellow PGDEPI
Professor
Padmashree Dr Vithalrao Vikhe Patil Foundation's
College of Physiotherapy
Ahmednagar, Maharashtra, India

Shyam Ganvir
BPhT MPhT PGDGC PhD Scholar
Principal, Professor and Head
Padmashree Dr Vithalrao Vikhe Patil Foundation's
College of Physiotherapy
Ahmednagar, Maharashtra, India

JAYPEE The Health Sciences Publisher
New Delhi | London

Jaypee Brothers Medical Publishers (P) Ltd

Headquarters

Headquarters
EMCA House
23/23-B, Ansari Road, Daryaganj
New Delhi 110 002, India
Landline: +91-11-23272143,
+91-11-23272703
+91-11-23282021, +91-11-23245672
E-mail: jaypee@jaypeebrothers.com

Corporate Office
Jaypee Brothers Medical Publishers (P) Ltd.
4838/24, Ansari Road, Daryaganj
New Delhi 110 002, India
Phone: +91-11-43574357
Fax: +91-11-43574314
E-mail: jaypee@jaypeebrothers.com

Overseas Offices

J.P. Medical Ltd
83 Victoria Street, London
SW1H 0HW (UK)
Phone: +44 20 3170 8910
Email: info@jpmedpub.com

EU GPSR Authorised Representative
Logos Europe, 9 rue Nicolas Poussin
17000, La Rochelle, France
Phone: +33 (0) 6 67 93 73 78
E-mail: Contact@logoseurope.eu

Website: www.jaypeebrothers.com

Website: www.jaypeedigital.com

Manual Therapy Approaches in Neurophysiotherapy

First Edition: 2016
Reprint: **2025**
ISBN 978-93-5090-964-5
Printed in India

Dedicated to

The loving memory of my mother Smt Lata M Jaipurkar
whose every effort was to see her children
repaying back to the society
and
this book is an attempt to do so

– Suvarna Ganvir

Preface

Manual therapy techniques are included in the third and final year physiotherapy syllabus by Maharashtra University of Health Sciences, Nashik, Maharashtra, for the last 10 years. But these students face difficulty in finding the resource material related to these techniques. The books which are available on these techniques are either not easily accessible to the students or if they are available, they are too elaborative, usually meant for therapists or for postgraduate students. Being undergraduate students, it is not possible for them to make a gist of the techniques really needed for their level. In an attempt to do so, many important points related to the techniques are missed.

Hence, there was a need for a comprehensive book, which would give an overview of these important techniques meant for effective treatment of patient suffering from neuromuscular superimposed or secondary musculoskeletal conditions. This book is an attempt to introduce the students to these techniques. A brief yet meticulous explanation of each technique is given. The sequence of description has followed a common pattern of definition, principles, technique, most important effects and uses of each technique. Considering it to be practical-oriented approaches, every effort is made to give examples of each procedure with detailed explanation. For further clarification of commonly used procedures, photographs depicting them are given. This book is by no way a replacement to the literature related to these approaches which are the results of the hardwork of all the stalwarts in the field of manual therapy. This is a tiny attempt to help the students better comprehend these approaches.

We hope that students find this book to be useful to understand the manual therapy techniques. We would also appreciate if the teachers would consider this book to be a constructive and handy adjunct for their regular teaching.

Suvarna Ganvir
Shyam Ganvir

Contents

CHAPTER

1

Introduction to Approaches

An examination or evaluation is performed by the physiotherapist before intervention to establish the objective measurements, to help diagnose functional limitations and impairments as well as to determine the prognosis of the outcomes based on the patients potential for functional improvement motivation, family support, financial support and cultural biases and to guide selection of various treatment strategies.

Using current motor learning, motor control theories, and systems models, the therapist must also determine the flexibility, and/or inherent motor control that the patient demonstrates while execution of the functional activities. During evaluation phase the therapist must break down the components of movement and must determine which if any is causing distortions or inefficient execution of the overall plan. The therapist must examine analyze, and diagnose the strengths and limitations of the client's motor system. Motor analysis must also cover the environmental, ethical and social contexts. Functional goals must be established that lead to the client's control over his/her environment and whenever possible lead to or maintain the quality of life desired by the client.

When selecting treatment interventions the therapist must differentiate between somatosensory retraining, functional retraining and augmented facilitatory treatment interventions. All three methods can be used simultaneously but the therapist needs to determine which aspect of the intervention falls into which methodology.

The challenge to educated professional is to determine what is being done why it is working, how to continue and how to determine the progress of the successful intervention. The professional must also determine how to empower the client to take over the intervention with inherent automatic mechanisms that lead to fluid, functional, flexible outcomes independent of both the therapist and the environment within which the activity is occurring.

Physiotherapy professionals are specialists in the analysis of movement with the scientific background to understand why the movement is occurring, what the strengths and limitations are within the system to support that movement and how different types of interventions can facilitate different types of intervention can facilitate functional movement strategies that ultimately carry over into functional life activities. Physiotherapists are also knowledgeable about neurological and organ system diseases and how progression of these pathological states affect motor performance and quality of life as well as about assistance and support needed to help clients maintain functional skills during transitional disease states. Similarly, therapists are currently taught how to minimize impairments within the sensory and motor system before functional loss. Early intervention before disability can prevent further or full function.

Hence to select an appropriate technique is a challenge to budding professionals. Before one select a technique for any condition, it is utmost important to know the basic principles of each technique. The knowledge regarding the procedure of conduct of each technique is imperative to its effective implementation. Each technique has a central condition in which, it is most effective. But its application in certain other conditions opens new areas of research, which is essential for the development of profession.

In the subsequent chapters, the reader will be exposed step-by-step to the recent techniques used in the management of patients with neuromuscular conditions. It is desirable that the readers use this information as baseline knowledge for effective practical implementation. Each technique is preferably described under common headings such as definition, principles, technique of application, effects and uses. Principles are mainstay for every techniques around which practical application revolves. Technique of application of each approach is explained in requisite details which will make it easy for the reader to apply on frequently seen patients. Effects will help the readers to identify the potential candidates for the application of any approach.

To treat patients with neuromuscular diseases, selection of appropriate treatment approach is essential. Research has indicated that a combination of treatment approaches may prove to be more effective than a single approach. Clinical signs and symptoms are the best indicators for selecting an approach or a combination of approaches. Any approach works to its best if the indications for the same are given due consideration. When patients are being given treatment it is imperative that due respect is given to the discomfort or pain that the patient is experiencing. Sometimes the ideal position for a particular technique is not possible. In that case, it the therapist's duty to select near ideal position for giving the treatment. Patients with neurological dysfunction may also have an additional other system involvement which might force to modify the selected treatment approach. For example, patients with stroke with hemiparesis may have a musculoskeletal dysfunction in the form of shoulder pain with a possible condition called shoulder-hand syndrome. In such a case even though it is indicated to use PNF technique, it may not be possible in the presence of pain. Hence individual discretion in selecting the appropriate approach will yield desired effects.

Duration and frequency of the selected approach will depend on the severity of the condition as well on the present functional level of the patient. At times the therapy needs to be administered twice a day or thrice a day, but usually once in a day is sufficient to get the desired effects. This will be maximally effective only when there is a functional carryover throughout the day. Any approach will lose its effectiveness if patient does not practice the learnt motor behavior during his daily activities. Hence, psychological counseling of the patient to persuade motor behavior that was learnt as a part of any approach into the functional activities throughout the day. For example, if during the treatment patient is taught to stand-up from sitting position by partially bending forward to keep the COG forward, then he should make use of this strategy, every time he gets up from sitting position, throughout the day. If he fails to do so, the effectiveness of any approach gets nullified.

Further, it is necessary to quantify the effect of this approach on functional recovery in patients with various neurological disorders. Hence, it is always recommended to use specific outcome measures to detect the improvement in any condition as a response to these therapeutic techniques. Details of these outcome measures are given as an appendix in the end. Psychometric properties of these measures is proven in the available literature and hence can be used liberally in the conditions specified and otherwise also.

Before one learns about approaches it is necessary to know regarding the different theories of motor learning and motor control that forms the basis of these approaches. These theories must be applied practically during implementation of various approaches.

THEORIES OF MOTOR CONTROL

Motor control is the ability to regulate or direct the mechanisms essential to movement. It addresses the questions such as, how does the central nervous system organize many individual muscles and joints into coordinated functional movements? How is the sensory information from the environment and the body used to select and control movement? What is the best way to study movement? How can movement problems be quantified in patients with motor control problems?

Why should We Study Motor Control?

We are referred as applied motor control physiologists. This is because therapist spends considerable amount of time retraining the patients who have motor control problems producing functional movement disorders. Therapeutic interventions are often directed at changing the movement or capacity to move. Therapeutic strategies are to improve the quality and quantity of postures and movements essential to function. Thus understanding the motor control and specifically the nature and control of movement is critical to clinical practice.

Nature of Movement

Movement emerges from the interaction of three factors: the individual, the task and the environment. The individual generates movement to meet the demands of the task being performed within the specific environment. The individual's capacity to meet interacting task and environmental demands determines that person's functional capability.

Individual Considerations

Movement arises from the interaction of multiple processes including those that are related to perception, cognition and action.

Movement and action: It is often described within the context of accomplishing a particular action. As a result, motor control is usually studied in relation to specific actions or activities. Understanding the control of action implies understanding the motor output from the nervous system to the body's effectors systems or muscles. The body is characterized by a high number of muscles and joints, all of which must be controled during the execution of coordinated, functional movement. This problem of coordinating many muscles and joints has been called the degrees of freedom problem.

Movement and perception: Perception is essential to action just as action is essential to perception. Perception is integration of sensory impressions into psychologically meaningful information. Sensory perceptual systems are provide, information about the state of the body and features, within the environment critical to regulation of movement. Therefore, sensory/perceptual information is clearly integral to the ability to act effectively within the environment. Thus, understanding movement requires the study of systems controling perception and the role of perception in determining our actions.

Movement and cognition: In addition since movement is not usually performed in the absence of intent, cognitive processes are essential to motor control. Motor control includes perception action systems, that are organized to achieve specific goals or intents. Thus, the study of motor control must include the study of cognitive processes as they relate to perception and action.

Task constrains on movement: In everyday life, we perform a tremendous variety of tasks requiring movement. The nature of the task being performed in part determines the type of movement needed. Thus understanding the control of movement requires an awareness of how tasks regulate or constrain movement.

Recovery of function following CNS damage requires that a patient develop movement patterns that meet the demands of functional tasks in the face of sensory/perceptual, motor or cognitive impairments. Thus, the therapeutic strategies that help the patient learn or relearn to perform functional tasks are essential to maximizing recovery of functional independence. Within clinical environment, tasks are routinely grouped into functional categories. Examples of functional task groupings include bed mobility tasks, transfer tasks, etc.

Classification based on task attributes: Tasks are classified based on the understanding of the essential attributes of a task that specifically govern or regulate the control of movement.

Discrete versus continuous tasks a critical attribute of a discrete movement tasks is a recognizable beginning and end. Kicking or throwing a ball, moving from sitting to standing and lying down. The end point in discrete is an inherent attribute of the task itself and cannot be arbitrarily defined by a performer. In contrast to discrete movements, continuous movements have no recognizable beginning or end point. A series of discrete movements that are performed together are referred to as serial movements. Serial movements while at first appearing continuous, are actually composed of an ordered series of discrete movements.

Stability versus mobility tasks, it is classified according to whether the BOS is still or in motion. Stability tasks are performed with a non-moving base of support. In contrast a feature or attribute of mobility tasks such as walking running is a moving base of support. Between these two ends are the tasks that entail more complex movements over a modified base of support such as moving from sitting to standing.

Manipulation continuum: Movement tasks are classified according to manipulation component. Manipulation tasks that require both speed and accuracy increase the demands on the postural system, since stabilization of the body is critical to the performance of these tasks.

Attention continuum tasks that have lowest attentional demands are primarily static postural tasks, attention demands increase in mobility tasks.

Open versus closed tasks: An essential attribute of open movement tasks is variability and flexibility, since they are performed in unpredictable environments. Open movement tasks are performed in a constantly changing environment, making the ability to plan a movement difficult. Closed movement tasks are characterized by fixed habitual patterns of movement with minimal variation. They are performed in a relatively fixed environments. While open movement tasks vary greatly from trial to trial in response to changing environmental features, closed movement tasks are relatively stereotyped, showing little trail-to-trail variations. Because of stereotypical nature of closed movement patterns they have lower information processing and attentional demands than open movement tasks which place greater demands on the information processing systems.

Environmental constraints on movement: To be functional CNS must consider the attributes of the environment when planning task specific movement. Attributes of the environment that affect movement have been divided into regulatory and nonregulatory features. Regulatory features specify aspects of the environment that shape the movement itself. Nonregulatory features of the environment may affect the performance, but movement does not have to conform to these features. Features of the environment in some instances enable or support performance or alternatively disable or hinder performance. Thus understanding features within the environment that both regulate and affect the performance movement tasks is essential to planning effective intervention.

Three levels of analyzing the movement, a part of clinical practice is analyzing, how and why patients move the way they do/Gentile suggested that goal directed functional behavior can be analyzed at three levels action.

Action: It examines the behavioral outcome that results from the interaction of the individual, the task and the environment.

Movement level: Focuses on analyzing the movements used to perform the functional tasks.

Neuromotor level: Movement can be analyzed from the perspective of the underlying process that contribute to the movement being performed. It also means analysis of subsystems of movement, both individually and collectively.

Theories of motor control: A theory of motor control is a group of abstract ideas about the control of movement. A theory is a set of interconnected statements that describe unobservable structures or processes and relate them to each other and to observable events. Jules Henri said science is built up of facts, as a house is built of stone; but an accumulation of facts is no more a science than a heap of stones is a house. A theory gives meaning to facts, just as a blueprint provides the structure that transforms stones to a house.

Value of theory to practice: Actions of therapists are based on assumptions that are derived from theories. Thus motor control theory is a part of the theoretical basis for clinical practice. Theories provide the following: a framework for interpreting the behavior, a guide for clinical action. New ideas, working hypotheses for examination and intervention.

Frame work for interpreting behavior: Theories help therapists to interpret behavior or actions of patients they work with. Theory allows the therapist to go beyond the behavior of one patient and broaden the application to a much larger number of cases. When a theory and its associated assumptions does not provide an accurate interpretation of a patients behavior, it loses its usefulness to the therapist. Thus, theory have a potential to limit a therapist's ability to observe and interpret movement problems in patients.

Guide for clinical action: Theories provide therapists with a possible guide for action. Clinical interventions designed to improve motor control in patients with neurological dysfunction are based on an understanding the nature and cause of normal movement and an understanding of the basis of abnormal movement. Therapeutic strategies aimed at retraining motor control reflect this basic understanding.

New ideas: Dynamic and evolving theories are dynamic, and they change to reflect greater knowledge relating to the theory. Expanding theories can broaden and enrich the possibilities for clinical practice. New ideas related to examination and intervention will evolve to reflect new ideas about the nature and cause of movement.

Working hypothesis for examination and intervention: A theory is not directly testable since, it is abstract. Rather theories generate hypotheses which are testable. Information gained through hypothesis testing is used to validate or invalidate a theory. This same approach is useful in clinical practice. So called hypothesis driven clinical practice transforms the therapist into an active problem solver. Using this approach to retrain the patient with motor dyscontrol calls for the therapist to generate multiple hypotheses.

Reflex theory: Sir Charles Sherrington formed the experimental foundation for a reflex theory of motor control. For Sherrington reflexes were the building blocks of complex behavior. He believed that reflexes worked together or in sequence to achieve common purpose. The conception of a reflex requires three structures, a receptor, a conducting nervous pathway and an effector. He stated that with nervous system intact, the reaction of the various parts of that system, the simple reflexes, are combined into greater actions that constitute the behavior of individual as a whole.

Limitations: (1) The reflex cannot be considered as the basic unit of behavior if both spontaneous and voluntary movements are recognized as acceptable classes of behavior since the reflex must be activated by an outside agent. (2) The reflex theory of motor control does not adequately explain and predict movement that occurs in absence of a sensory stimulus. (3) Sherrington does not explain fast movements that is sequences of movements that occur too rapidly to allow for sensory feedback from the preceding movement to trigger the next. (4) The reflex chaining model fails to explain that a single stimulus can results in varying responses depending on the context and descending commands. (5) Reflex chaining does not explain the ability to produce novel movement.

Clinical implications: If chained or compounded reflexes are the basis for functional movement, clinical strategies designed to test reflexes should allow therapist to predict function. In addition patient's movement behaviors would be interpreted in terms of the presence or absence of controling reflexes. Finally, retraining motor control for functional skills would focus on enhancing or reducing the effect of various reflexes during motor tasks.

Hierarchical theory: Hughlings Jackson states that the brain has higher middle and lower levels of control equated with higher association areas the motor cortex and spinal levels of motor function. Hierarchical has in general been defined as organizational control that is top down. That is, each successively higher control exerts control over the level below it. This theory suggests that motor control emerges from reflexes that are nested within the hierarchical organization levels of the CNS. Normal motor development was attributed to increasing corticalization of CNS resulting in the emergence of higher levels of motor control over lower level reflexes. This has been called Neuromaturational theory of development. Modern neurosciences have confirmed importance of elements of hierarchical organization in motor control. The concept is a strict hierarchy in which higher centers are always in control, has been modified. Current concepts describing hierarchical control within the nervous system recognize the fact that each level of nervous system can act upon other levels depending on the task. Also reflexes are not considered the sole determinant of motor control but only one of the many processes important to the generation and control of movement.

Limitations: One of the limitation of this theory is that it cannot explain the dominance of reflex behavior in certain situations in normal adults.

Clinical implications: It is used widely in the treatment of the conditions such as stroke to describe the disordered movement following a motor cortex lesion. When the influence of the higher centers is temporarily of permanently interfered with normal reflexes become exaggerated and so called pathological reflexes appear. With cerebral palsy the theory is explained as the release of motor responses integrated at lower levels from restraining influences of higher centers, especially that of a cortex leads to abnormal postural reflex activity.

Motor programming theory: The concept of central motor pattern or motor program is more flexible than the concept of reflex because it can be activated either by sensory stimuli or by central processes. It states that movement is possible in the absence of reflexive action. Sensory input, while not essential in driving movement has an important function in modulating action. Central pattern generators (spinally mediated motor programs) by themselves can generate such complex movements. Central pattern generator is a specific neural circuit.

Limitations: Central motor program cannot be considered to be the sole determinant of action. The motor program concept does not take into account the fact that the nervous system must deal with both musculoskeletal and environmental variables in achieving movement control.

Clinical implications: Motor program theory have allowed clinician to move beyond a reflex explanation for the disordered motor control. Explanations of abnormal movement have been expanded to include problems resulting from abnormalities in central pattern generators and in higher level motor programs. In patients whose higher levels of motor programming are affected motor program theory suggests, the importance of helping patients relearn the correct rules for action. In addition intervention should focus on retraining movements important to a functional task not just on re-educating specific muscles in action.

Systems theory: During the course of any movement the amounts of force acting on the body change as potential and kinetic energy change. The same central command can result in quite different movements because of the interplay between external forces and variations in the initial conditions. According to this theory coordination of movement is the process of mastering the redundant degrees of freedom of the moving organism. The higher levels of nervous system activate lower levels, the lower levels activate synergies or groups of muscles that are constrained to act together as a unit. Bernstein believed that synergies play an important role in solving the degrees of freedom problem. This is achieved by constraining certain muscles to work together as unit. He hypothesized that there are few synergies; they make possible almost the whole variety of movements.

Limitations: It does not focus heavily on the interaction of the organism with environment.

Clinical implications: It stresses the importance of understanding the body as a mechanical system. Movement is not determined solely by the output of the nervous system but is the output of the nervous system filtered through a mechanical system, the body. When working with the patient who has a CNS deficit, the therapist must be careful to examine the contribution of impairments in the musculoskeletal system to overall loss of motor control.

Dynamic action theory: It says that when a system of individual parts comes together its elements behave collectively in an ordered way. There is no need for a higher center issuing instructions or commands to achieve coordinated action. This principle applied to motor control predicts that movement can emerge as a result of interacting elements without the need of specific commands or motor control programs within the nervous system. Dynamical theory suggests that the new movement emerges because of a critical change in one of the systems called a control parameter. A control parameter is a variable that regulates a change in the behavior of the entire system. Attractor stated may be considered preferred patterns of movement used to accomplish common activities of daily life. The degree to which there is a flexibility to change a preferred pattern of movement is characterized by as an attractor well. The deeper the well the harder, it is to change the preferred pattern, suggesting a stable pattern. A shallow well suggests an unstable pattern. It is also shown that stable movement patterns become more variable or unstable just prior to the transition to a new movement pattern.

Limitations: It presumes that the nervous system has a fairly unimportant role and that the relationship between the physical system of the animal and environment in which it operates primarily determines the animal's behavior.

Clinical implications: Shifts or alterations in behavior can be explained in terms of physical principles rather than necessarily in terms of neural structures.

Ecological theory: The ability to use perceptions to guide action emerges early in life. Perception focuses on detecting information in the environment that will support the actions necessary to achieve the goal. From an ecological theory point of view, it is important to determine how an organism detects information that in environment that is relevant to action, what form this information takes, and how this information is used to modify and control movement.

Limitations: It gives less emphasis to the organization and function of the nervous system, which led to this interaction.

Clinical implications: The active exploration of the task and the environment in which the task is performed allow the individual to develop multiple ways to accomplish a task. Adaptability is important not only in the way we organize movements to accomplish the task but also in the way we use the perception.

THEORIES OF MOTOR LEARNING

Motor learning is defined as the study of the acquisition and/ or modifications of movement. While motor control focuses on understanding of the control of movement already acquired motor learning focuses on understanding the acquisition and/or modification of movement. The field of motor learning has traditionally referred to stud of acquisition or modification of movement in normal subjects. In contrast, recovery of function has referred to the acquisition of movement skills lost through the injury.

Early Definitions of Motor Learning

Learning has been described as the process of acquiring knowledge about the world; motor learning has been described as a set of processes associated with practice or experience leading to relatively permanent changes in the capability for producing skilled action. This definition of motor learning reflects four concepts.

a. Learning is the process of acquiring the capability for skilled action.
b. Learning results from experience or practice.
c. Learning cannot be measured directly; instead it is inferred from behavior.
d. Learning produces relatively permanent changes in behavior; thus short-term alterations are not termed as learning.

Broadening the Definition of Motor Learning

It emerges from a complex of perception–cognition-action process. Now the process of learning can be described as the search for a task solution that emerges from an interaction of the individual with task and environment. Task solutions are new strategies for perceiving and acting. Similarly, the recovery of function entails the reorganization of both perception and action systems in relation to specific tasks and environment.

Relating performance and learning: Thus learning defined as a relatively permanent change has been distinguished from performance defined as a temporary change in motor behavior seen during practice sessions. Performance whether observed during practice sessions or during retention and transfer tasks, is the result of complex interaction amongst many variables, only one of which is level of learning.

Forms of learning: The recovery of function following injury entails the acquisition of complex tasks. However, it is difficult to understand the processes involved in learning using the study of complex tasks. Hence, we will look at simpler aspects first moving towards the complex aspects.

Nonassociative forms of learning it occurs when animals are given a single stimulus repeatedly. As a result the nervous system learns about the characteristics of that stimulus. Habituation is a decrease in responsiveness that occurs as a result of repeated exposure to a nonpainful stimulus. Sensitization is an increased responsiveness following a threatening or a noxious stimulus.

Associative forms of learning: It involves association of ideas. It is through associative learning that a person learns to predict relationships of one stimulus to another (classical conditioning) or the relationship of ones behavior to a consequence (operant conditioning). Patients who have injury that has drastically altered their ability to sense and move in their world must reexplore their body in relation to their world to determine what new relationships exist between the two.

Classical conditioning: Consists of learning to pair two stimuli. During classical conditioning an initially weak stimulus becomes highly effective in producing a response when it becomes associated with another stronger stimulus. It has recently been shown that we generally learn the relationships that are relevant to our survival; it is more difficult to associate biologically meaningless events. These findings underscore an important learning principle the brain is more likely to perceive and integrate aspects of environment that are most pertinent. With regard to therapy, learning in patients is most likely to occur in tasks and environment that are relevant and meaningful to them .

Operant Conditioning

It is basically trial and error learning. During this we learn to associate a certain response among many that we have made with a consequence. Behaviors that are rewarded tend to be repeated at the cost of other behaviors. Likewise behaviors that are followed by aversive stimuli are not usually repeated. This has been called the Law of effect. Using biofeedback to help the patient to learn to control the foot during swing phase of the gait is an example of operant conditioning.

Procedural and Declarative Learning

Procedural learning refers to learning tasks that can be performed without attention or conscious thoughts like a habit. Procedural learning develops slowly through repetitions of an act over many trials and is expressed through improved performance of the task. Procedural learning does not depend on awareness, attention or other higher cognitive processes. Declarative learning results in knowledge that can be consciously recalled and thus requires processes such as awareness, attention and reflection. The advantage of, that it can be practiced in other ways than it was learned. In therapy, when clinicians are helping the patients reacquire skills lost through injury, the emphasis is often on practices leading to procedural learning rather than on declarative learning. Declarative learning requires the ability to express verbally the process to be performed and is often not possible for the patients who have cognitive and language deficits that impair their ability to recall and express knowledge. Teaching movement skills declarative does however allow patients to rehearse their movement mentally, increasing the amount of practice available to them when physical conditions such as fatigue otherwise limit it.

THEORIES OF MOTOR LEARNING

It is a group of abstract ideas about the nature and cause of the acquisition and or modification of movement.

Adam's Closed Loop Theory

Adams a researcher in physical education was the first person to attempt to create a comprehensive theory of motor learning. The most important concept was a closed loop process in which a sensory feedback is used for the ongoing production of skilled movement. The idea was that in motor learning, sensory feedback from the ongoing movement was compared with in the nervous system with the stored memory of intended movement. This theory also propose two distinct types of memory, the first called memory trace was used in the selection and initiation of movement. The second called perceptual trace was built over a period of practice and became the internal reference of correctness. He proposed that after movement is initiated by memory trace, perceptual trace carry over to complete the movement and detect error.

Clinical implications: Learning a new movement skill with practice gradually a perceptual trace is developed for the movement that serves as a guide for later movement. The more the patient practices a movement, the more perfect the perceptual trace becomes. In fact, the accuracy of movement is directly proportional to the strength of perceptual trace.

Limitations: Animals and humans can make movements even when they have no sensory feedback. Animals are capable of certain types of learning even after sensory deaffrentation. The closed theory cannot explain the accurate performance of a novel movement or of open loop movements made in the absence of sensory feedback. Memory storage process within the brain would make it impossible to store a separate perceptual trace for every movement ever performed. Finally variation in the movement practice may actually improve motor performance of task more than practicing moving to a single end point.

Schmidt's Schema Theory

It emphasised on open loop control processes and the generalized motor program concept. Schmidt predicted that when learning a new motor program, the individual learns a general set of rules that can be applied to a variety of contexts. At the heart of this motor learning theory is the concept of schema. The term schema originally referred to an abstract representation of stored in memory following a multiple presentations of a class of objects. Generalized motor program is considered to contain rules for creating the spatial and temporal patterns of muscle activity needed to carry out a given movement. Schmidt proposed that after an individual makes a movement four things are stored in a memory.

a. Initial movement conditions such as the position of the body, weight of an object manipulated
b. The parameters used in a generalized motor program
c. Outcomes of movements in terms of knowledge of results
d. The sensory consequences of movement.

The recall schema is used to evaluate the response. When the movement is over the error signal is fedback into the schema and the schema is modified as a result of sensory feedback and KR. Thus according to this theory, learning consists of a ongoing process of updating the recognition and recall schemas with each movement that is tried.

Clinical implications: Optimal learning occurs if the task is practiced in under many conditions. This allows patient to develop a set of rules for teaching which can be applied when reaching for a variety of glasses or cups. As rules for reaching improve, patient will become more capable of generating appropriate reaching strategies for picking up an unfamiliar glass with less likelihood of dropping the glass or spilling the milk.

Limitations many studies show large effects of variable practice while some studies show very small effects or no effects at all. Another limitation is that it lacks specificity. Because of its generality, few recognizable mechanisms can be tested. Thus, it is not clear how schema processing itself interacts with other systems during motor learning and how it aids the control of movement. Another challenge ot schema theory is its inability ot account for the immediate acquisition of new types of coordination.

Ecological Theory

Newell suggests that motor learning is a process that increases the coordination between perception and action in a way consistent with the task and environmental constraints. He proposes that during practice there is a search for optimal strategies to solve the task, given the task constraints. There is a search for the optimal perceptual cues as well thus both perception and action systems are incorporated or mapped into an optimal task solution. Exploring the perceptual workplace requires exploring all possible perceptual cues to identify those that are most relevant to the performance of a specific task. Perceptual cues that are critical to the way in which a task is executed are called regulatory cues. Perceptual information related to understanding of the goal of a task and the movements to be learnt. Perceptual information also gives feedback both during the movement (concurrent feedback) and on completion of movement (knowledge of results). Finally it is proposed that perceptual information can be used to structure the search for a perceptual motor solution that is appropriate for the demands of the task. Thus in this approach, motor learning is characterized by optimal task relevant mapping of perception and action, not by a rule based representation of action.

Clinical implications: It suggests patients learn to distinguish the relevant perceptual cues important to organizing action. Also during recovery of motor skills, an important part of motor learning is learning to discriminate between relevant and irrelevant perceptual cues. Knowledge of the critical perceptual cues associated with a task is essential in dealing with a new variation of the task. When faced with a novel variation of the task the patient must actively explore the perceptual cues to find information necessary to solve the task problem optimally.

Limitations: One of the major limitations is that it has yet to be applied to specific examples of motor acquisition an any systematic way.

THEORIES RELATED TO STAGES OF LEARNING MOTOR SKILLS

Another set of theories look at motor learning from a motor temporal perspective. These theories begin by describing initial stages of acquisition and describe how learning occurs over time.

Fitts and Posner three stage Model

They suggest that there are three stages involved in skill learning. In the first stage the learner is concerned with understanding the nature of the task, developing strategies that can be used to carry out the task and determining how the task should be evaluated. These efforts require a high degree of cognitive activity such as attention hence called as cognitive stage of learning. Second stage is associate stage wherein refinement of skill takes place. There is less variability in performance improvement also occurs slowly. It is proposed that verbal cognitive aspects of learning are less important in this stage because person focuses more on refining a particular task. This stage may last days to weeks or months depending on the performer and intensity of practice.

Third stage is called the autonomous stage wherein, there is automaticity of the skill and the low degree of attention required for its performance. Thus in this stage the person can begin to devote his/her attention to other aspects of skill in general.

Clinical implications: When first learning a new task, it would require a great deal of attention and conscious thought. When moving towards the second stage, the task is refined as the person develops optimal strategy. In the third stage the person would be able to carry out the task with varied environmental constraints or simultaneously involved in other task.

Systems Three Stage Model

The emphasis is on controlling the degrees of freedom as a central component of learning a new movement skill. When a novice is learning a new skill the degrees of freedom of the body are constrained as they perform the task to make the task easier to perform. As the task is gradually mastered the learner begins to release the degrees of freedom and learns to coordinate the movements at two or more joints, which allows for more movement efficiency freedom and thus skill. Vereijken et al used this approach to develop a model of the stages of motor learning. They suggest the first stage of motor learning is the novice stage in which the learner simplifies the movement to reduce the degrees of freedom. They suggest that this is accomplished by constraining or coupling multiple joints together so they move in unison and by fixing the angles of many joints involved in movement. These constraints are made at the cost of efficiency and flexibility in response to changing task or environmental demands. The second stage called the advanced stage is the one in which the performer begins to release additional degrees of freedom by allowing more movements at more joints involved in the task. Simultaneous contraction of agonist and antagonists at a joint is reduced and muscle synergies across a no of joints are used to create a well coordinated movement that is more adaptable to task and environmental demands. The third stage, called the expert stage, is one in which the individual now has released all the degrees of freedom necessary to perform the task in the most efficient and best coordinated way. In addition the individual has learned to take the advantage of the mechanics of the musculoskeletal system and of the environment and to optimize the efficiency of the movement.

Clinical implications: It suggests the possible explanation for the co-activation of muscles during the early stages of acquiring a motor skill and as an ongoing strategy for patients who are unable to learn a motor control a limb dynamically. Alternatively motor development could be viewed from a biomechanical perspective as gradual release of degrees of freedom. Finally this theory suggests the importance of providing external support during the early phases of learning a motor skill in patients with coordination problems. Providing external support constraints the degrees of freedom that the patient initially has to learn to control. As coordinative abilities improve, support can be systematically withdrawn as the patient learns to control more and more degrees of freedom.

Limitations: Very little research is focused on the autonomous stage of learning, partly because it would take months or year as to bring many subjects to this skill level on a laboratory task. Thus, the principle that govern motor learning processes that lead to this stage of mastery are largely unknown.

Gentile's two Stage Model

In the first stage the goal of the learner is to develop an understanding of the task dynamics. At this stage learners are just getting the idea of the requirements of the movement. This includes understanding the goal of the task, developing movement strategies appropriate to achieving the goaland understanding the environmental features critical to the organization of them movement. At this stage one learns to distinguish relevant regulatory features of the environment from those that are nonregulatory. In the second stage called the fixation/diversification stage, the goal of a learner is to refine the movement. Refining a movement includes both developing the capability of adapting the movement to changing tasks and environmental demands and performing tasks consistently and efficiently. The terms fixation and diversification refer to the distinct requirements of open versus closed skills. Closed skills have minimal environmental variations and thus require a consistent movement pattern with minimal variation. In contrast, open skills are characterized by changing environmental conditions and therefore require movement diversification.

BIBLIOGRAPHY

1. Anne Shummway-cook, Marjorie H Woollacott: Motor Control Theory and Practical Applications. 2nd edn. Lippincott Wiliams Wilkins, 1992.
2. Bobath B. Adult Hemiplegia: Evaluation and Treatment. 3rd edn. London, UK: William Heinemann Medical Books; 1990.
3. Carr J, Shephard R. Neurological Rehabilitation: Optimizing Motor Performance. Oxford, United Kingdom: Butterworth-Heineman; 1998.
4. Gentile AM. Skill acquisition: action, movement and neuromotor processes. In: Carr JH, Shepherd RB, (Eds). Movement Sciences: Foundation for Physical Therapy in Rehabilitation. 2nd edn. Gaithersburg: Aspen; 2000.
5. Ryerson SD, Umphred DA, Neurological Rehabilitation 3rd edn. St Louis, Mo: CV Mosby Co; 1995.

CHAPTER

2

Bobath Technique

Learning Objectives

At the end of chapter the learner shall be able to:

1. Define the terms associated with this approach.
2. Describe the synergy patterns in upper and lower extremities.
3. Describe six foundations of the technique.
4. Describe the basic techniques used.

Berta Bobath, a physical therapist, and her husband Dr Karel Bobath have developed a special method of treatment commonly used in the treatment of patients with adult hemiplegia. It is most effective when used by the entire health care team in the 24 h/day care of the physiotherapy. The principles of treatment can be followed by all those concerned with the case. It is ideal to begin treatment immediately during the acute stages of illness but effective treatment can be started at any time.

This technique is mainly evolved for the patients with lesions of upper motor neurone such as hemiplegic and cerebral palsy. The main problem of these patients is that of abnormal coordination of movement patterns combined with abnormal postural tonus. Problems of the strength and activity of the individual muscles or muscle groups we see as that of secondary to that of the coordination. There is a lack of control of muscle function. Muscles are the end organs of the nervous system and hence the activity of the individual muscles and muscle groups is secondary to that of their coordination in patterns of activity. Thus, the assessment and treatment of the patient's motor problem is the only way of leading directly to functional use. In the patients with hemiplegia muscles are not paralyzed and deficits of muscular activity can be remedied by their action in more normal functional patterns. Holistic approach is needed for better patient management. It should take care of sensory, behavioral and perceptual problems of the patient.

The patient's main problem is his inability to direct the nervous impulses to his muscles in many varied ways and in the different combinations of patterns used by a person with an intact central nervous system. The main task of treatment is that of improving tonus and coordination by obtaining normal active reactions of the affected side in response to being moved. Normal reactions to being moved indicate the patient's ability to perform same movements independently and voluntarily.

The patient's more normal reactions to being moved during treatment shows his potential and are a guide to the therapist in planning treatment. They also show which techniques to use and not to use and how to use them, all this depending on the patient's responses throughout the treatment. It is important to monitor these responses for better or worse by a constant feedback between the patient and therapist. Heavy resistance exercises, irradiation and the use of associated reactions should be avoided in patients with spasticity as it will reinforce the existing released tonic reflexes, and with it, increases the spasticity. Following the flaccid stage, patients enter a stage of mixed tone, displaying a combination of flaccidity and spasticity for, e.g. the upper extremity might have an increased tone proximally and a reduced tone distally.

Spasticity is the most common and most difficult motor problems to treat following CVA. If not treated correctly, spasticity can progress to a point so that independent living is nearly impossible. Spasticity interferes with the patient's ability to move by interfering with selective motor function. It produces abnormal sensory feedback and contributes to weakness of the antagonistic even when there is no actual affection in the muscles. It can cause contractures, pain and fear in many patients; pain, fear and spasticity are often so intermixed that a vicious circle appears. Thus musculoskeletal problems are superimposed on the primary neuromuscular problems. The spasticity can cause an increase in pain on stretching such tightened structures which can cause an increased fear which in turn increases the amount of spasticity.

If measures are taken to reduce pain and fear the therapist has a much better chance for success with the methods used to reduce spasticity. The typical posture of the adult hemiplegic patient is a combination of strongest components of flexion and extension synergies.

Trunk: Lateral flexion toward the involved side with rotation away from the involved side.

i.e.	Scapular	-	Depression, retraction
	Shoulder	-	Adduction, internal rotation
	Elbow	-	Flexion
	Forearm	-	Pronation
	Wrist	-	Flexion and radial deviation
	Fingers	-	Flexion

Trunk: Lateral flexion toward the involved side, trunk shortening

i.e.	Pelvis	-	Postelevation, retraction
	Hip	-	Internal rotation, adduction, extension
	Knee	-	Extension
	Ankle	-	Plantar flexion, supination and inversion
	Toes	-	Flexion

The one fortunate characteristic about spasticity is the fact that it can be influenced. This means that the therapists can reduce or inhibit the effects of spasticity to some degree.

The patient's main problem is his inability to direct the nervous impulses to his muscles in many varied ways and in the different combinations of patterns used by a person with intact central nervous system. The main task of treatment is that of improving tonus and coordination by obtaining normal active reactions of the affected side in response to being moved. Normal reactions to being moved indicate the patient's ability to perform the same movements independently and voluntarily.

In the patient with spasticity more normal coordination cannot be achieved as long as tonic reflexes are active, evidenced by the abnormal postural patterns of extensor and flexor spasticity. Since spasticity is not confined to the any one muscle group, but to the synergy patterns, inhibition of these patterns reduces spasticity and this can be done by the therapist changing and dissociating the spastic patterns. However, without the patient being active while the therapist changes a position, there is no carryover of this inhibitory action into his own and unassisted movement. The patient has to learn to control actively the widespread patterns of spasticity.

Inhibition of those parts of the movement, which are unnecessary and might interfere with a specific activity produces a great variety of motor responses which enable the normal person to perform manual skills. The hemiplegic patient not only lacks the necessary variety of motor patterns, but is also unable to combine various patterns. For instance, he will be able either hold or manipulate an object which is lying on a table but he will not be able to hold and manipulate it at the same time or when the arm is lifted up. The main problem in performing skilled movements is their complexity. They need constantly changing combinations of easier and less selective movements, which are a part of the more complex combinations which constitute a skill.

Normalization of movements can be accomplished by using one or more of the following techniques:

1. **Proper positioning:** The patients should be properly positioned especially in the acute stage. The upper extremity is positioned by the side of the body with elbow in extension and wrist joint in neutral position. Different positioning is needed for patients with or without extensor spasticity in the lower extremities. The flexor tendency in lower limbs is dangerous for rehabilitation. Therefore, the therapist must prevent flexion contracture in the hip and knee joints.
2. **Weight-bearing over the affected sides**: Weight bearing enhances awareness of joint position sense by stimulating the proprioceptors present in the joints (Fig. 2.1).

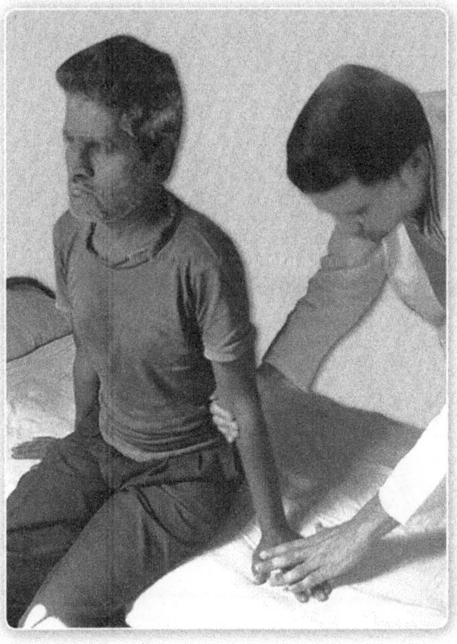

Fig. 2.1: Showing weight-bearing on upper extremity

3. **Trunk rotation**: several things occur as patient rotates the trunk. Rotation encourages weight bearing and elongation of the affected side provides a vestibular input. Through trunk rotation the patient not only helps to normalize the movements tone but also learns to better integrate both sides of the body (Fig. 2.2).
4. **Elongation of the trunk in the affected side:** It helps in working towards the symmetry of the trunk. This can be accomplished in lying, sitting and standing positioning. The use of reflex inhibiting patterns and prolonged stretch is that it not only reduces tone in the proximal regions but also has an effect distally as well (Fig. 2.3).
5. **Shoulder protraction:** It accomplishes two goals. (a) It helps to normalize the movement tone (b) It helps to maintain scapular mobility. When the patient pulls back in scapular retractions an increase in tone in the flexor pattern can be detected throughout the upper extremity. Shoulder protraction is an effective method of reducing flexor tone in upper extremity (Fig. 2.4).

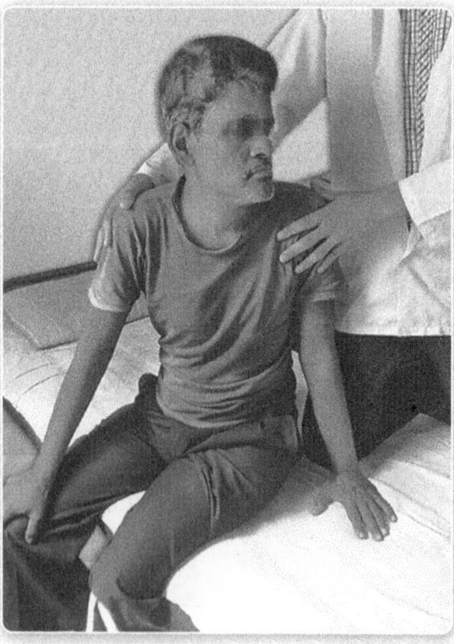

Fig. 2.2: Showing trunk rotation activities

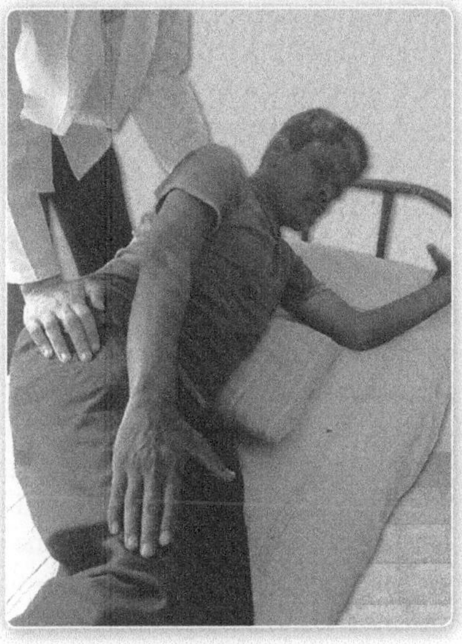

Fig. 2.3: Showing elongation of the trunk in the affected side in lying position with the affected side down

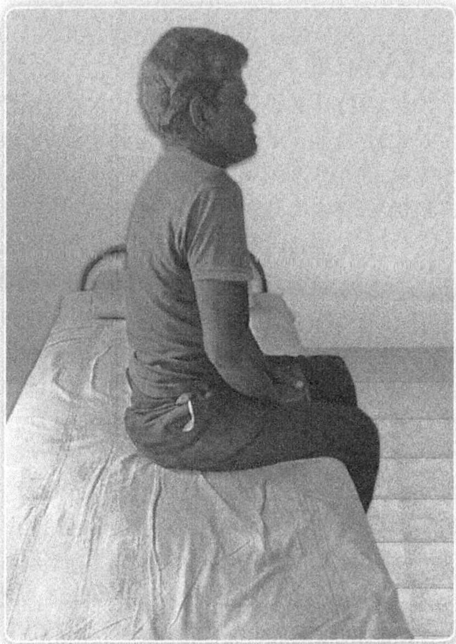

Fig. 2.4: Showing shoulder protraction exercises

6. **Careful gradation of stimulation:** Stimulation can refer to a number of things. Auditory stimulus affects muscle tone. The therapist's voice, background noise or any loud noise can produce an in increase in tone. Tactile stimulation can also increase or decrease the muscle tone depending on how and length of time it is applied. Stimulation can also be the rate of an activity or facilitation techniques is performed.

These are six points provide foundation for treatment of adult hemiplegic using Bobath approach. The techniques are most effective and provide the best potential in the rehabilitation when they are started in acute phase at the time of admission in the hospital. These techniques however can be used in any phase of recovery.

Short-term rehabilitation in the hospital saves time and has economical advantages. However even after discharge from the hospital, the patient needs further treatment for a prolonged period in the put patient department or at home. If the potential recovery of the affected side and its treatment is taken into consideration right from the beginning and throughout the whole time of the patient's treatment, his rehabilitation will not take longer and the results will be better.

The usual aim of treatment during the early and acute stages of adult hemiplegic is that of short-term rehabilitation with a view of getting the patient out of the bed and making him as independent as possible in the activities of daily living. In order to get him to walk as soon as possible the emphasis of treatment is placed on the sound side in compensation for loss of the affected side. He is given a tripod on which to lean, which brings his whole weight to the sound side and make him use his sound leg for balance and walking. As he cannot bend his knee and ankle, he has to use his trunk to help him bring the affected leg forward to make a step, causing him to hitch-up his pelvis. The leg is stiff and is used momentarily as a prop to carry his weight, most of which is taken on a tripod or elbow crutch or later on a stick. The patient is taught also, to use his sound arm and hand for self help, for pushing and pulling himself upto sitting for getting out of bed for standing up from the chair, etc. This program of compensatory rehabilitation is usually supplemented with exercises to strengthen the muscles and to maintain joint ranges.

Even after the discharge from the hospital once the acute stage is over, patient needs further treatment for prolonged time period in the outpatient department or at home. If the potential recovery of the affected side and its treatment is taken into consideration from the beginning and throughout the whole time of treatment, his rehabilitation will not take longer and results will be better.

The aim of treatment should be to inhibit the patient's abnormal patterns of movement. One cannot superimpose normal over abnormal. They should be reinforced and perpetuated by the effort involved in strengthening the muscles. The movements, the patient performs with or without the therapists help should not be done with undue effort. Effort leads to increase in spasticity and produces widespread associated reactions. Heavy resistance exercises, irradiation, use of associated reactions and mass synergies should be avoided in patients with upper motor neurone (UMN) lesion. In UMN lesions the tonic reflexes are disinhibited and dominant to the total. Exclusion of every other pattern of coordination. The influence of tonic reflexes is present in normal persons and produces slight and transient tonus changes among the wealth of many other postural and movement patterns. But in spastic conditions if disinhibited, the use of effort, irradiation and mass movement patterns of tonic reflexes to strengthen the muscles will only reinforce the existing released tonic reflexes and with it increase the spasticity.

It has been found ineffective to use static reflex inhibiting postures. Although, the spasticity becomes reduced temporarily, there is no carryover into the patient's own functional activity. If he attempts to move independently, spasticity returns immediately as he can only use the total spastic patterns. The therapist has to help him to use only parts of total pattern and prevents reassertion by her handling. The patient is encouraged and enabled to use parts of total pattern selectively. While he moves, the therapist prevents, i.e. inhibits the unwanted parts of the abnormal total pattern. It is the restoration of this inhibitory control that makes the permanent reduction of spasticity possible and gives him selective movements and their various combinations of functional skills. By learning to inhibit unwanted spread of activity throughout the affected parts of the body, he controls associated reactions. This process is called autoinhibition.

Initial Flaccid Stage

Treatment started in early stages should help the patient to carry weight on the affected side and to learn to balance on the affected side in sitting and standing. It should also help in working bilateral function of arms and trunk, so that the required interplay of the sound side with affected side becomes possible.

The commonly employed techniques during this stage are positioning and moving of the hemiplegic patients. Patients should be so positioned that it should inhibit unnecessary flexor and extensor tone in upper and lower extremity respectively. Patients are trained to turn on their affected and normal side. Being able to use the bedpan is the next goal of treatment. This is followed by making the patient to sit up at the edge of bed from normal as well as affected side. Once the patient is able to sit, he is taught to balance himself in sitting position.

Stage of Spasticity

There is always some overlap between acute stage and second stage. In this stage, most of the treatment would be done in sitting and standing. breaking up of all the patterns is now needed for better adaptation of movements to functional 7 selective skills. No separation of arm or leg activity should be made permanantly. Lack of balance and difficulty in moving the affected leg in walking will increase the flexor spasticity in the arm and hand. Also effort and abnormal walking will prevent any potential use of the arm. Decrease in spasticity of the trunk and arm will decrease the extensor spasticity of the leg and make easier. This also allows more normal movements of the leg is possible in standing and walking.

Stage of Relative Recovery

The patients, who reach the third stage of relative recovery will be those who were not severely affected at the beginning and who have made a good spontaneous recovery, or who have done well in the treatment. These patients now will be able to walk unaided, i.e. may be without using a stick. They may, however, be unable to use the hand for manipulation or have difficulty in doing so. It is desirable that these patients, who are able to work and to lead an independent life in the community, should be further helped by improving the quality of their gait and by obtaining a better use of their affected hands.

Spasticity is minimal at this stage and does not therefore prevent movement. Transient increase of spasticity, however still occurs when the patient uses effort, walks fast, or gets excited; coordination then deteriorates.

Treatment to Improve Patient's Gait

If further improvement in the patient's gait is to be achieved, it is necessary to obtain still more selective movement of his knee and of dorsiflexion and plantar flexion of ankle and toes, independent of the position and movement of the hip. Full dorsiflexion of ankle and toes is essential for normal walking and for heel toe strike.

Crossed standing and walking is another way of improving, his balance and control of his hips, and is a preparation for rotation of the pelvis in walking. It also helps turning round toward the sound side, which the patient finds difficult as he cannot bring the affected side sufficiently forward.

When walking the therapist is at the patient's affected side. His arm is held in external rotation and extended by his side slightly diagonally backwards. His wrist and fingers should be extended and his thumb abducted. Walking can also be practiced with the therapist behind the patient, holding both arms backwards as described when sitting on a stool. Rotation of the shoulder girdle should also be practiced in standing. He swing arms from side-to-side rotating his trunk and touching the opposite thigh with one hand. To practice the same movement when walking the therapist stands in front of the patient and holds him by both hands while she walks backward. Another, and even better, way of introducing rotation into the patient's walking pattern can be done by the therapist standing behinx d him and rotating his hips and shoulder girdle.

BIBLIOGRAPHY

1. Berta Bobath: Adult Hemiplegia: Evaluation and Treatment, 2nd edn. Heinmann Medical books,1978.
2. Raine S. Defining the Bobath Concept using the Delphi technique. Physiother Res Int. 2006;11:4–13.
3. Lennon S. The Bobath Concept: a critical review of the theoretical assumptions that guide physiotherapy practice in stroke rehabilitation. Phys Ther Rev. 1996;1:35–45.

CHAPTER

3

Brunnstrom's Approach

Learning Objectives

At the end of the chapter, learner shall be able to:
1. Describe recovery stages according to Brunnstrom.
2. Describe basic limb synergies.
3. Describe basic components of this approach.
4. Describe the procedure of treatment to be followed at each component.

RECOVERY STAGES ACCORDING TO BRUNNSTROM

Stage 1: Immediately following acute episode, flaccidity of the involved limbs is present and no movement, on either a reflex or voluntary basis can be initiated.
Stage 2: As recovery begins the basic limb synergies or some of their components may appear as associated reactions, or minimal voluntary movement responses may be present. Spasticity begins to develop and may be particularly evident in muscle groups that dominate synergy movements.
Stage 3: The patient gains voluntary control of the movement synergies although the full range of synergy components does not necessarily develop. Spasticity which may become severe in some cases reaches its peak. This stage in the recovery process may be thought of as semi-voluntary in that the patient is able to initiate the movement in the involved limbs on a volitional basi but is unable to control the form of resulting movement, which will be the basis of limb synergies.

Stage 4: Some movement combinations that do not follow the paths of basic limb synergies are mastered, first with difficulty, then with increasing ease. Spasticity begins to decline, but the influence of spasticity on nonsynergistic movements is still readily observable.
Stage 5: If recovery continues more difficult movement combinations are observed as the basic limb synergies lose their dominance over the motor acts. Spasticity continues to decline.
Stage 6: Individual joint movement becomes possible and coordination approaches normalcy. As spasticity disappears, patient becomes capable of a full spectrum of movement patterns.
Stage 7: As the last recovery stage, normal motor function is restored.

BASIC LIMB SYNERGIES

Normal movement is characterized by synergistic motor behavior, that is the coupling together of muscles in an orderly fashion as a means by which purposeful movement is achieved with maximal precision and minimal waste of energy. The basic limb synergies seen in patients with CVA are almost stereotyped and do not permit different combinations of movements. The group of muscles constituting a hemiplegic limb synergy acts together as a bound unit of motion and in the early stages of recovery following a CVA produces the same outcome irrespective of the patient's attempt to vary the outcome. The resultant movement, whether evoked volitionally or reflexly, are primitive, automatic, reflexive highly similar among all patients with hemiplegia, and reflect the loss of inhibitory control normally exerted by the higher centers of CNS integration.

Each of the limb synergies—two for upper, two for the lower limb—incorporate specific movement components regardless of whether the synergy is elicited reflexly or performed voluntarily by the patient.

Flexor synergy in the upper limb: If complete range of all components materializes, this synergy consists of the following: Retraction and/or elevation of the shoulder girdle, external rotation of the shoulder, abduction of the shoulder to 90°, flexion of elbow to an acute angle, full range supination of the forearm. The dominant component of the flexor synergy is elbow flexion, wherein elbow flexors display the greatest degree of spasticity in this pattern. The movement pattern is typically initiated by either elbow flexion or shoulder girdle elevation, with subsequent recruitment, to greater or lesser degree of the remaining components.

Extensor synergy of the upper limb: It has following components: fixation of the shoulder girdle in a protracted position, internal rotation of the shoulder, adduction of the arm in front of the body, extension of the elbow, complete range, full range pronation of the forearm. Shoulder adduction and internal rotation dominate the movement within the extensor synergy and if the movements are successful forearm pronation almost invariable comes into play. Extension of the wrist with fist closure often appears with extensor synergy but is by no means universal. Finger extension is not seen in either synergy; it does not generally appear until the influence of the synergies is on the decline.

Flexor synergy of the lower limb: The components are as follows: flexion of the hip, abduction and external rotation of the hip, flexion of the knee to about 90°, dorsiflexion and inversion of the ankle, dorsiflexion of the toes.

The flexor synergy is typically THE WEAKER of the two lower extremity synergies and is dominated by hip flexion. Owing to the influence of tonic reflexes, patients find it difficult to perform the flexor synergy in supine position but may succeed in accomplishing the movement, particularly hip flexion and ankle dorsiflexion in sitting position.

Extensor synergy in lower limb: The components are as follows: extension, adduction and internal rotation of hip, extension of knee, plantarflexion and inversion of ankle, plantar flexion of toes.

The extensor synergy typically dominates in lower extremity with considerable hip adduction, knee extension and ankle plantarflexion appearing. The synergy can almost be initiated through activation of the strongest component, knee extension. The quadriceps tends to be the most spastic component, but it is the adductor muscles that, strongly linked to the quadriceps in synergy interfere greatly with performance of upright activities.

Influence of postural reflexes: The attitudinal reflexes become easily demonstrable in the presence of certain types of pathology of nervous system. Their influence on the ability to perform voluntary movement may be so strong that a patient may be able to perform voluntary flexor and extensor movements only by utilizing the facilitating effect of one or the other of these reflexes. When a conflict between will and inhibitory reflex impulses exists, the will does not always gain supremacy.

Associated reactions: In patients with hemiparesis, reflex tensing of muscles and involuntary limb movement are frequently observed. These responses are known as associated reactions. In most patients voluntary forceful movements in other parts of the body readily elicits such reactions in the affected limbs. In the upper limb, the reactions are of the same type as the movements employed to evoke the responses, that is, flexion tended to evoke flexion and extension tended to evoke extension. Whereas in lower limb, the reaction of the opposite type to the movement employed to evoke the responses. Also, an associated movement may be evoked in a limb that is essentially flaccid, although latent spasticity may be present. Associated movements may occur in the affected limb under a variety of conditions: In the presence of spasticity, when the patient has achieved degree of ice voluntary control of the limb movements and after spasticity has essentially subsided. Associated movements may be present years after the onset of hemiplegia. Repeated stimuli may be required to evoke a response. Tension in the muscles of the affected limb decreases rapidly after cessation of stimulus that had evoked associated reaction. Attitudinal reflexes influence the outcome of the associated reactions.

Patients are assessed with respect to hand, upper extremity trunk and lower extremity. Gross testing of sensory loss concentrates mainly on patient's ability to recognize movements of the affected limbs, localization of touch in the hand and appreciation of pressure in the sole of foot.

Passive motion sense shoulder, elbow, forearm and wrist—with patient in sitting, the affected UL is supported by the investigator and moved to different positions while the patient observes the movement and performs identically on the unaffected limb. To begin with procedure has to perform on large joints and then small joints of hand can be checked. also patient can be asked to determine without looking as to which is lightly touched with rubber end of pencil. Passive motion sense, lower limb motor tests; shoulder and elbow.

They are preferably tested in sitting position. But if trunk control is not fair enough as in recovery stage 1 and 2, patients may be tested in supine position.

Recovery Stage

Recovery stage	Test	Hand
1	Heavy upper and lower limbs on passive movement, no active contraction is present	Flaccidity
2	Appearance of basic limb synergies, or some of their components on active contraction	Little or no finger flexion
3	Flexor synergy: "try to reach to your ear" Extensor synergy: "to touch the palm of the examiner's hand held between the patient's knees"	Mass grasp, use of hook grasp but no release; no voluntary finger extension; possibly reflex extension of digits
4	Placing the hand behind the body elevation of the arm to a forward horizontal position pronation, supination, with elbows flexed at 90°	Lateral prehension, release by thumb movement ; semivoluntary finger extension, small range
5	Arm raising to a side horizontal position Arm raising forward and overhead Pronation supination, elbow extended	Palmar prehension; possibly cylindrical and spherical grasp, awkwardly performed with limited functional use; voluntary mass extension of the digits, variable range
6	Speed tests	All prehensile types under control; skills improving ; full range voluntary extension of digits; individual finger movements present, less accurate than opposite side

Speed tests: These tests are specifically used in stages 4 to 6. For purposes of comparison, both the affected and nonaffected sides are tested. These tests closely resemble the flexor extensor synergy. The two tests are (with the patient in sitting position):

1. The hand is moved from lap to chin, requiring complete range of flexion of elbow.
2. The hand is moved from lap to opposite knee, requiring full range of extension of elbow.

   A stopwatch is used and the number of full strokes completed in 5 seconds is recorded, first on the normal and then on affected side. If the speed is slow, as would be the case when there is marked spasticity, half strokes are counted as well. These two tests give information concerning spasticity of flexor and extensor muscles of the elbow.

Motor Tests of Trunk and Lower Limbs

Recovery stage	Test
1	Flaccidity
2	Minimal voluntary movements of the lower limbs
3	Hip knee ankle flexion in sitting and standing
4	Sitting knee flexion beyond 90° with the foot sliding behind on the floor; voluntary dorsiflexion of the ankle without lifting the foot off the floor
5	Standing isolated non weight bearing knee flexion, hip extended, standing isolated dorsiflexion of ankle
6	Standing, hip abduction beyond range obtained from elevation of pelvis; sitting reciprocal action of inner and outer hamstring muscles, resulting in inward and outward rotation of the leg at the knee, combined with inversion and eversion of the ankle.

Treatment

Bed posture: It is recommended that whenever a patient of hemiplegia lies in the bed, slight hip and knee flexion should be maintained by a small pillow under the knee, lateral support of the knee should be given to prevent abduction and external rotation of the hip. Flexed hip and knee position is recommended as knee flexion though slight has an inhibitory effect on the extensor muscles of knee and ankle. In case if the flexor synergy predominates in the lower limb, it is advisable to keep hip and knee in some amount of flexion. The upper limb is supported on a pillow in a position with shoulder in slight abduction and wrist in slight extension.

Bed exercises: Passive movements followed by active assisted movements should be given. Also patients must be taught to go into side-lying position. Movement on the affected side is much easier as compared to on the Rationale for upper limb treatment "given that the stages of recovery are a normal sequence of events, it is further postulated that volitional control, or at least partial control, of the basic movement synergies is a prerequisite to the development of more advanced patterns and, ultimately more extensive motor control. That is to say, since a stage in the recovery process is not passed over, voluntary initiation of basic synergistic patterns of movement is encouraged as a means of achieving normal movement in both its quantitative and qualitative aspects.

The overall resemblance between normal motor development and recovery following a cerebrovascular accident is noted previously. While normal developmental milestones are achieved in a progressive manner, they are not perfected in their entirety before attempts at sequentially more advanced milestones are made. Each stage in the recovery process following a cerebral vascular accident may similarly be considered as a developmental milestone, one that is to be achieved but not perfected before attempting activities that characterise the next higher stage, but no stage is mastered before attempts at next stage are introduced. In general, assuming that the patient presents with flaccidity, background tension is developed using associated reactions or attitudinal reflexes or a combination thereof. Volitional effort is then superimposed on the reflexely produced background tension. When the patient is able to initiate movement on a voluntary basis, reflex assistance is withdrawn and movement patterns that deviate from synergy are introduced. During the synergy stages, patient is trained to use the affected arm as an aid to the normal arm. The extensor synergy may be used for the activities such as stabilizing an object while the unaffected arm is used to open an envelope or holding a bottle when the unaffected hand is opening the lid. The flexor synergy can be used for the activities such as to carry a briefcase or hand bag after the handles have been placed in the hand. During stages 4 and 5, voluntary effort enables the patient to learn a number of comparatively easy movement combinations that deviate from the basic synergies and then proceed to the more difficult combinations. Activities such as hand to chin, hand to ear, hand to opposite elbow, hand to opposite shoulder, etc. can be practiced at an early stage. These require grading of intensity of various flexor components. In some cases, wherein spasticity is more and any voluntary effort results in increased synergy pattern, hold after positioning technique is superior as an initial step towards achieving active movement through the desired range. The patients hand is placed in a desired position and then he is asked to hold the position. When the patient is able to hold the position slight lengthening contraction is initiated, then shortening contractions through increasingly larger ranges of movement, until the patient can successfully perform the movement through its entire range. It is followed by dissociation of the components of synergy pattern.

Hand Training

For hand to be effective the linkage between the muscles that hold wrist in extension and those that flex the digits, which is disturbed due to cerebral vascular accident, needs to be restored. In the early training the wrist is placed in the position of extension, with elbow in extension. One of the technique is, the patient is asked to flex his fingers thereby allowing eccentric contraction of wrist extensors. Alternately the wrist can be stabilized in extension passively followed by tapping over the wrist extensor muscles that acts as the reinforcement. Then the patient is asked to squeeze his fingers gently. Then the patient is further asked to slowly lower his wrist down thus activating the eccentric contraction of wrist extensors.

Besides this the patient is trained for stabilizing the wrist for the different activities of hand with elbow in different positions. Also spasticity in the flexor group makes release of the grasp difficult and hence this needs to be trained simultaneously. The commonly employed techniques are: the thumb is pulled out of the palm by a grip around the muscles of thenar eminence and the forearm is supinated passively, rapid passive finger flexion movements without interruption, elevation of the arm above the horizontal position and thereby evoking tonic extensor reflexes of the digits. When the extensor reflex of the digits is well established, the arm is passively lowered and the elbow is flexed with forearm and wrist supported. This is followed by alternate active finger flexion and release. Following this, voluntary opening of the fist is trained with the arm held in the elevated position. Once the patient masters the technique in this position, then he can be further trained to achieve wrist extension in different positions of the arm (Fig. 3.1).

Walking Training

Preparation for walking should include training in trunk balance, both sitting and standing; modification of motor responses of the limbs to

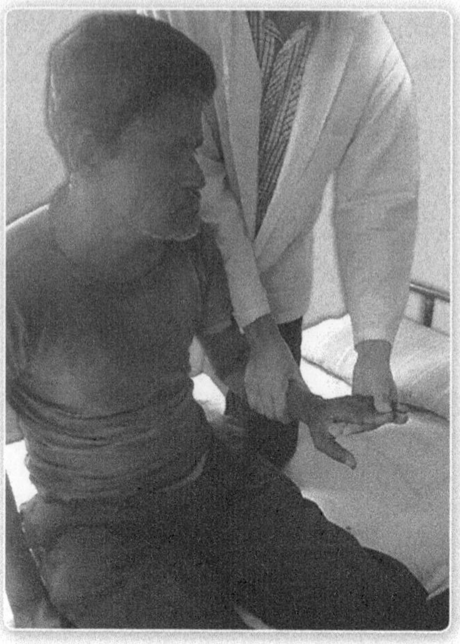

Fig. 3.1: Picture showing training of wrist extensors

obtain muscular associations resembling those that required for normal walking and training of alternate responses of antagonistic muscles to promote a rapid release in tension of muscle groups following their activatation.

- **Trunk balance:** This can be achieved in sitting by giving different trunk movements in different directions like bending forward or obliquely forward or bending sideways. If the patient's trunk balance is very poor, the therapist may use her own knees to stabilize the patient's knees, because the knee on the affected side has a tendency to fall into abduction. Besides other movements stated above patient can also be trained for trunk rotation in sitting position so as to increase the area of operation with upper extremity or lower extremity. For this initially the therapist guides the movement by holding the patient at the trunk and later on allowing the patient to do on his own (Fig. 3.2).
- **Modification of motor responses of the lower limb:** With the patient in sitting position, he can be asked to bend backward slowly to activate bilateral hip flexor muscles in an eccentric way. These muscles may also

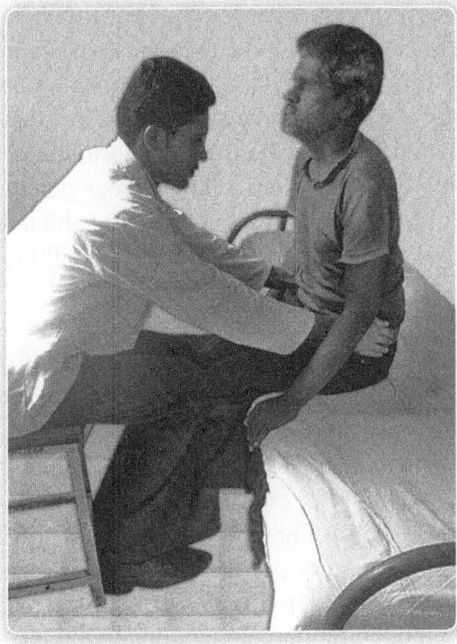

Fig. 3.2: Trunk balance training, therapist supporting the knees of patient

be activated with attempts to maintain the trunk erect against resistance. For unilateral contraction of hip flexor muscles, immediately following a trunk backward inclination, patient is asked to flex the hip. Further patient can also be encouraged to do dorsiflexion of ankle with hip flexion as both the movements are closely associated with each other. This association is called as 'Coordination synkinesis' by Marie and Fox (1916). Dorsiflexion can also be trained in different position of leg such as with knee flexion, with knee extension. Further dorsiflexion can also be associated with eversion of foot for proper gait.

In general, following rules for the recruitment of the muscles are followed:

- If voluntary control is not present in any position or movement combination, a contraction is elicited reflexely. The patient superimposes the voluntary effort on the reflex contraction. Local facilitatory measures are introduced to reinforce the patient's voluntary effort. Attempts are made to cause the muscle groups that have been activated to respond in the desired muscle action.

- For activation of the hip abductor muscles initially in supine position bilateral resistance to hip abductor muscles is applied with the hips in adduction for stretch reflex. Once the patient makes voluntary effort for hips abduction on the affected side, resistance is withdrawn suddenly. After few repetitions in this position progression can be made to side lying position, with vigorous percussion on gluteal muscles. Following this passive position of abduction is given and patient is asked to hold this position. This will help the patient to build up the reflex tension in the muscle.
- For bilateral activation of abductor muscles in standing position, with the patient in parallel bar, patient is asked to bear weight on the normal side and abduct the affected side. Then the opposite movement is done. In this if there is sagging of the pelvis on the affected side then manual support can be given to the affected side pelvis. Patient is further encouraged to bear more weight through the affected extremity. For unilateral action of hip abductor muscle in standing position the patient is asked to elevate the pelvis on unaffected side, enough to lift the foot on that side off the ground.

- **Alternate responses of antagonistic muscles:** Inability of the spastic muscles to release their tension rapidly and at proper time adversely affects all coordinated activities and markedly impairs locomotion. For training knee flexor muscles in supine lying position, local stimulation of the tendons of hamstring muscles or manipulation of soft tissues on the posterior side of thigh helps to release the tension. Patient can be asked to flex his knees completely followed by gradual heel sliding to full extension. With the patient in sitting position, he can be asked to flex the knee joint further making an acute angle with the thigh. this can be achieved by sliding the heel backwards. Knee flexor muscles can be further activated in half prone position. Patient can be asked to flex and extend his knee in this position irrespective of the position of hip joints. This half prone position can also be used for combination of movements such as knee flexion with plantar flexion and knee extension with dorsiflexion as required during the push off phase of gait. This combination of movements is called as 'Pawing'.

Standing and Walking

Stability of knee joint is most important for antigravity position which is equally challenging in patients with hemiplegia. For this patient must learn to bear weight through the affected side at least momentarily on the flexed knee joint. This can be achieved partially by alternate flexion and extension of the knee joint in standing position.

Trunk Rotation with arm Swing

Patients with hemiplegic tends to walk with inadequate trunk rotation and if spasticity is present in upper limbs, with elbow flexed and shoulder immobilized. Hence trunk rotation can be trained in sitting position with arms folded across the chest. But in standing position, the arms can be hung sideways. Trunk rotation in standing is a part of advanced training and good balance is a pre-requisite. The routine arm swing is absent in these patients. To encourage it, passive positioning of the arm is done as the patient takes a step forward. Thus, if a patient takes a step forward on the left side there occurs left rotation and therapist assists the patient to take the right hand forward as a swing .

Assisted Walking

Initially patient can be taken in parallel bars but use of parallel bars should be kept to minimum. This is because when in the parallel the tendency to bear more weight on the unaffected side is continued. Also at times patient finds it difficult to hold the bar with affected hand and hence may be more fearful to imbalance. When inside the parallel bars, it is advisable for the therapist to walk along with the patient.

Independent Walking

When walking outside the parallel bars, the patient can be given assistance by the therapist. Patients usually walk with shuffle gait taking short steps with minimal knee flexion during swing phase. Some patients find it difficult to perform the shuffle gait. Instead, they walk with exaggerated hip flexion, as if to clear the obstacles in their path. Because of the synergistic relationship, exaggerated hip flexion helps activate the ankle dorsiflexors.

Obstacle Walking

This is advocated for those patients who tend to drag the foot on the affected side during swing phase. obstacles are placed in their path at regular intervals. Patient is instructed to lift the leg up so as to clear the obstacle placed in their way. A slow walking rhythm is maintained as the right and left foot step over the obstacles of equal height (Fig. 3.3).

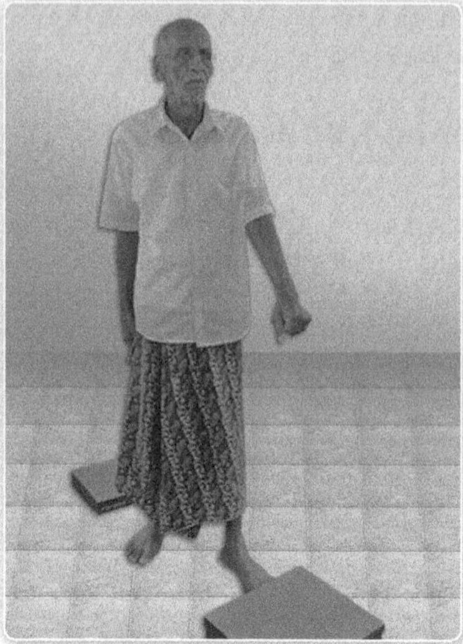

Fig. 3.3: Obstacle walking

Stairs

While climbing stairs, the unaffected foot leads in ascending while affected foot in descending. Patient may be allowed to take the support of a railing if he needs.

BIBLIOGRAPHY

1. Pedretti L, Early M. Occupational Therapy: Practice Skills for Physical Dysfunction. 5th edn., Mosby, London, 2001.
2. Sawner K, La Vigne J. Brunnstrom's Movement Therapy in Hemiplegia: A neurophysiological approach. 2nd end, JB Lippincott Company, Philadelphia, 1992.

CHAPTER

4

Neurodevelopmental Technique

Learning Objectives

At the end of the chapter the learner shall be able to

1. Define Neurodevelopmental technique (NDT).
2. Describe the principles of NDT.
3. Describe key concepts.
4. Explain the assumptions behind the approach.

INTRODUCTION

The neurodevelopmental technique (NDT) first known as "Bobath approach" was originated and developed by Dr Keral Bobath. It is an advanced hands-on approach to the examination and treatment of the individuals with disturbances of function, movement and postural control due to a lesion of central nervous system.

NDT is primarily based on the following principles:

1. Muscle tone can be reduced by the use of reflex inhibiting postures.
2. The treatment protocol ideally should consist of hierarchical motor sequence, i.e. from head control to rolling to quadruped to sitting to standing.
3. Automatic motor sequence is more facilitated more than isolated developmental skills.
4. It is a problem solving approach using a system or a selectionist model.
5. It is a distributed model of CNS structure and function.

6. Although, CNS is the controller, it functions determines the pattern of neural activity based on input from multiple intrinsic systems and extrinsic variables that establish the context of initiation and execution.
7. Sensory feed forward is equally important as that of feedback for different aspects of movement control.
8. Negative signs such as weakness, impaired postural control and paucity of movement needs to be balanced with positive signs such as limitations of function.

The basic philosophy is that lesions in CNS produce problems in the coordination of posture and movement combined with atypical qualities of muscle tone that contribute directly to the functional limitations. These functional limitations are changeable when the intervention strategies target specific system impairments in activities and contexts that are meaningful in the life of a person. It is used primarily for children with cerebral palsy (CP) but can also be used in patients with cerebrovascular accidents (CVA).

Following are the assumptions underlying the NDT approach:

1. Primary problems in children with CP are impaired patterns of postural control and movement coordination.
2. Treatment needs to directly address neuromotor and postural control abnormalities in the context of the task.
3. Missing or atypical elements that link functional limitation to system impairments are identified at the assessment. These are used as intervention strategies.
4. It is the whole individual who is affected by sensorimotor impairments, i.e. the person's function, place in the family and society, independence and overall functioning.
5. A working knowledge of typical adaptive motor development and how it changes across the life span provides the framework for assessing function and planning intervention.
6. NDT clinicians focus on changing movement strategies as a means to achieve the best energy-efficient performance for the individual within the context of the age appropriate tasks and in anticipation of future functional tasks.
7. Motor component is linked to sensory processing.
8. Active initiation and participation on the part of the patient forms important intervention strategies, often combined with therapist's manual guidance and direct handling.
9. Ongoing evaluation occurs throughout every treatment session.
10. The aim of NDT is to optimize function.

KEY CONCEPTS

1. The treatment approach should follow principles of normal motor development. The normal motor development usually follows a sequence, i.e. from cephalad to caudal, from proximal to distal, from gross to fine.
2. Feedback is closed a system, e.g. sensory-motor-sensory.
3. During normal development there is:
   a. Interplay between stability and mobility.
   b. Interplay between agonists and antagonists muscles during coordinated muscle movement-reciprocal innervations.
   c. Restoration of the head in vertical position during movements at other parts of the body—righting reactions.
   d. Maintenance or regaining of the balance during a shift in COG-equilibrium reactions.
   e. Development of the postural control in three planes.
   f. Dissociation of movement, i.e. certain movements can be performed in isolation.
4. Motor development follows a sequence.
5. Abnormal development occurs when there is a breach in above pattern.
6. Hence, sensory input is used to bring about a change in motor output.

The main focus of assessment is to identify the client's abilities and limitations in order to tailor an individualized treatment plan and provide a basis for comparing the client's abilities at a later point in time.

What differentiates NDT intervention from other approaches is the precise therapeutic handling, including facilitation and inhibition, used to provide sensoriomotor cues that facilitates change in function (Howle, 2004).

"Handling is graded input provided by the therapist's hands at key points of control on the child's body.... and results in active control or movement" (Kramer, 1993, p. 78).

The key points (proximal or distal) are the places of physical contact between the therapist's parts of the body or therapy equipment and client's body. (Boehme, 1988).

"Facilitation is the process of intervention which uses the improved muscle tone in goal-directed activity. Facilitation techniques involve stimulation of the muscle activity to produce a desired motor response. It is related with the functional goal that needs to be achieved."

"Inhibition is the process of intervention that reduces dysfunctional muscle tone."

Key principles used for enhancing the function through the approach are as following.

a. Set anticipated outcomes and impairment goals in partnership with the family, the client, and the interdisciplinary team.
b. Establish a treatment plan with anticipated outcomes that include specific, observable functions within a specific time frame under specific environmental conditions. Therapy utilizes client's strengths, recognizes that each individual has competencies and disabilities.
c. Treatment strategies often include preparation and simulation of critical foundational elements (task components) as well as practice of the whole task. It mainly includes planning and solving motor problems. They are repeated periodically which is an important component in any motor learning theory. Knowledge of the development of posture and movement components is use in designing treatment strategies.
d. Progression is done from simple to complex activities. A single treatment session progresses from activities in which the client is most capable to activities that are more challenging. Individual treatment sessions are designed to evaluate the effectiveness of treatment with the session.
e. NDT intervention methods include modifying the task, or the environment, and take into account the current level of the client's performance and capacity for function.
f. Families receive information regarding the client's problems and management of those problems, as they are able to understand and assimilate the information.
g. Considering the long duration of treatment an attempt is made to create an environment that is conducive to cooperative participation and support of the client's efforts. NDT recommends an interdisciplinary model of service. Coordinate with the goals and activities of all other medical, therapeutic, social, and educational disciplines to ensure a life-span approach to solving the client's problems.

The key points (proximal or distal) are the places of physical contact between the therapist's parts of the body or therapy equipment and client's body. (Boehme, 1988).

Proximal key points: These are located closer to the source of the problem, usually at the head, trunk, or large joints. They are used to influence posture and movement in all three planes (sagittal, frontal, and transverse), especially during difficult moment (Fig. 4.1).

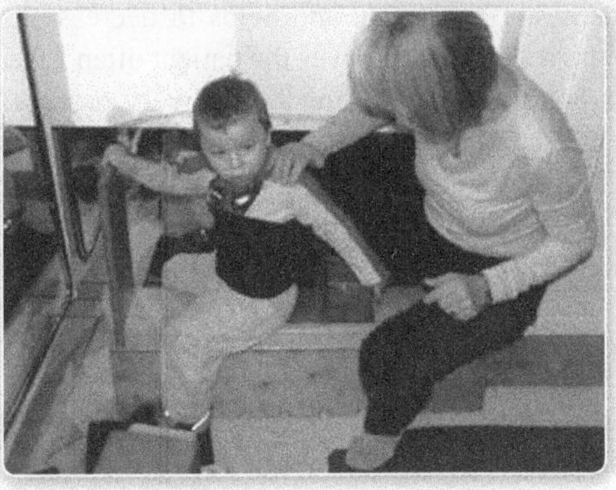

Fig. 4.1: Proximal key points

Distal key points: These are located away from the source of the problem, usually at the upper and lower extremities level. They are used to allow the client to engage in activities with minimal control of the therapist (Fig. 4.2).

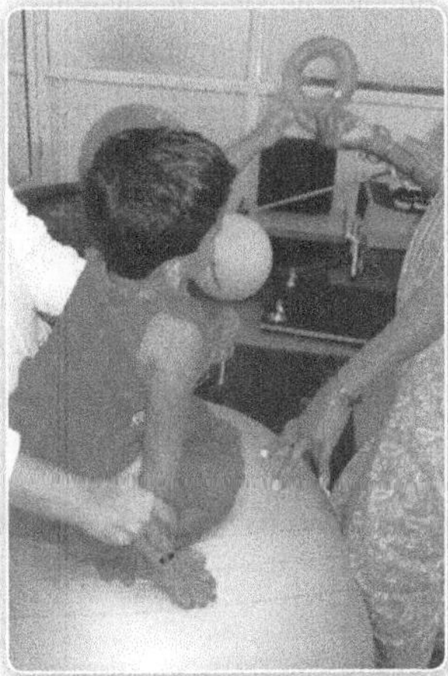

Fig. 4.2: Distal key points

WEIGHT-BEARING OVER THE AFFECTED SIDE

Weight bearing over the hemiplegic side is the most effective way of noramlizing tone. With patients displaying low tone it is facilitative and with patients high tone it can be inhibitory. Weight bearing not only helps normalize tone, it also provides sensory input to the hemiplegic side through proprioception. Additionally, this approach improves the patient's awareness of that side and helps to decrease neglect. As the awareness of the weak side improves the patient often is less fearful, thus establishing a better foundation for the recovery process. The positive effects of weight bearing can be observed in early stages of recovery. Correct weight bearing can be as simple as positioning. The patient should be taught to bear weight equally through both hips in sitting and both feet in standing.

TRUNK ROTATION

It is very effective way of normalizing tone and facilitating normal movement througth upper extrimity and lower extremity. Patients with hemiplegic often walk in a block pattern, with little separation of shoulder and pelvic girdle. To facilitate normal movement, the therapist should set-up activities to facilitate or stimulate trunk rotation, which activates trunk musculature and aids in trunk stability. Without trunk stabilization the patient will be unable to use the upper extremity effectively.

When facilitating trunk rotation in sitting or standing, take the opportunity to vary the height of the task. This approach helps to incorporate not only the rotational components of movement but mobilizes the shoulder and pelvic girdle and improves weight shift to the hemiplegic side. Additional benefits from activities facilitating trunk rotation include the following—increased sensory input to the hemiplegic side, improved awareness of the hemiplegic side and trained compensation for the visual-field defects.

Scapular protraction before trying to open clenched fingers, first bring the scapula into forward protraction. Do not pull the arm, instead gently cradle the arm while placing the other hand along the medial border of the scapulal and bring the scapula forward.

POSITION OF PELVIS

Sitting is the position which encourages abnormal posture resulting in increased hip extension and rounding of the upper thoracic region with resultant head and neck extension. This posture has an adverse effect on swallowing, impedes normal alignment of the scapula and humerus and encourages flexion synergy of the UE proper alignment of pelvis, shoulder and head position in sitting can be attained by bringing the pelvis forward into a more neutral position.

Facilitation of slow controlled movements—benefits the patients with high tone quick movements increase tone and tend to set off an associated reactions resulting in a flexion synergy of upper extremities. To be most effective in tone normalization, the patient must be taught to use slower more controlled movements.

PROPER POSITIONING

Abnormal postures manifested in flexion and extension synergies of the upper and lower extremities promote compensatory movement and should be avoided. In sitting, avoid excessive posterior pelvic tilt lower extremity, external rotation, asymmetry of the trunk and head and scapular retraction.

RATIONALE FOR USE OF NDT TECHNIQUE

The primary goals of NDT is to relearn normal movements. The technique used are intended for more than just the moves of an arm or leg, they treat the person as a whole, encouraging the use of both sides.

The Bobaths used specific principles to inhibit abnormal patterns of movement. This impression or inhibition of normal patterns synergies must be accomplished before normal selective is related movement can take place. It is impossible to super impose normal movement on a person with abnormal tone. The therapist develops a program to help the patient avoid these abnormal patterns of movement. The program provides a foundation that promotes the highest level of functional recovery based as relearning normal movement. Rather than on compensation.

One of the central principles of NDT is that alignment and symmetry of the trunk and pelvis are necessary for good alignment and symmetry of the extremities.

Adaptive equipment is used when absolutely necessary for safety but not as a first resort and not as a replacement for treatment.

The following terms are often used in desiring NDT technique of Bobath.

Positioning, rotation of trunk, placing, spasticity inhibition, weight-bearing scapulas mobility, normalization of tone, postural reactions, protective extension

Additional terms associated with this approach and their definitions are

Associated movements: Extraneous movements that occur normally are seen in children adults when new difficult tasks are performed learned. For example, child displays associated movements when cutting scissors, when he or she sticks the tongue in and out, the movements can also be the same types of movements of both limbs, the activity of the limb not involved in the motor task reinforces that of the limb on the opposite side of the body involved in the motor task.

Associated reactions: Activity that requires excessive effort of the unaffected limbs can result in apparent limb movements, usually in a synergy patterns as palpable in tone of the affected limbs. Associated reactions are abnormal and occur as result of tonic reflexes or released postural reactions in us as deprived of volume control. These reactions must be prevented in HT. The point should be careful when wing any part of his or her body excessive effort.

Key points of control: Points on the body usually proximal, e.g. shoulder and pelvic girdles when handled by the therapist in a specific manner can be used to change part of an abnormal pattern to normal mount through the body and to guide the patient's active movements spasticity of the limbs can be influenced and reduced from these key points of control.

POSTURAL TONE

Postural tone as defined by the Bobaths it is normal activation of large groups of movements in patterns for the maintenance of posture normal, postural tone is high enough to resist gravity and low enough to give way to movements.

Reflex inhibiting patterns: Patterns of movements are opposite to spastic patterns and guided by the therapist from key points of control are used to inhibit abnormal motor activity and facilitate more normal motor activity.

Motor Problems

The major problems in hemiplegia is the lack of postural control affecting volume movements flaccidity and most common at the onset of condition. During this time, the patient is often passive, displaying low endurance and low tolerance for activity. This may last a few days or as long as several months. Although the patient displays no movement affected extremities at this time, a proper treatment program can be a strong impact on the eventual functionally outcome.

BIBLIOGRAPHY

1. Boehme R. Improving upper body control. An approach to assessment and treatment of tonal dysfunction. Tucson, AZ: Therapy Skill Builder. 1988.
2. Howle JM. Neuro-develompmental treatment approach. Theoretical foundations and principles of clinical practice. Laguna Beach, CA: NDTA. 2004
3. Ottenbacher KJ, Biocca Z, DeCremer G, Jedpvec KB, Johnson, MB. Quantitative analysis of the effectiveness of paediatric therapy: emphases on the neurodevelopmental treatment approach. Physical Therapy. 1986;66: 1095–101.

CHAPTER

5

Rood Approach

Learning Objectives

At the end of the chapter, the learner shall be able to

1. Identify the basic assumptions related to the technique.
2. Describe the principles of treatment.
3. Elaborate sequence of motor development.
4. Enlist components of ontogenic motor patterns.
5. List and describe various facilitation and inhibitory techniques.

In the year 1950 Rood devised a technique developed for facilitation and inhibition of movement through various stimuli.

BASIC ASSUMPTIONS

Motor Output is Dependent upon Sensory Input

Motor response follows a normal developmental pattern and psychic somatic and autonomic functions are interrelated.

Rood combined controlled sensory stimulation with a sequence of positions and activities of normal ontogenic motor development to achieve purposeful muscular responses. Thus, according to Rood muscle action could be activated, facilitated and inhibited through the sensory system.

Normalize Muscle Tone

Patients with neurologic dysfunction may have muscle tone ranging from hypotonic to hypertonic. Normalized muscle tone flows smoothly and is constantly changing during a motor act. The demands placed on different muscle groups are different. Hence, Rood said muscles have different duties, i.e. light work and heavy work. The light work muscles (mobilizers) are primarily flexors and adductors used for the skilled movement patterns. The heavy work muscles (stabilizers) are primarily extensors and abductors used for postural support.

Treatment Begins at the Developmental Level of Functioning

The patient is evaluated developmentally and treated in a sequential manner. The patient does not proceed to the next level of sensorimotor development until some measure of voluntary control is achieved. This principle follows a cephalocaudal rule.

Movement is Directed towards Functional Goals

Neurologically the pyramidal system is used to control reflex activity and to perform isolated voluntary acts. However, the coordination of the agonist muscles, antagonists muscles and synergies is a function of the extrapyramidal system. Complex motor patterns rely on subcortical centers for modification and correction, so that the cortex can concentrate on the purpose of the act. In addition, when the patient performs a willed movement with an intended goal, more neurons throughout the nervous system must discharge to initiate the task.

Repetition is Necessary for the Re-education of Muscular Responses

Thousands of repetitions are required for formulation of "engrams". Engrams are interneuronal circuits involving specific neurons and muscles to perform a pattern of motor activity. To avoid monotonicity similar motor patterns add purpose and value to the exercise.

PRINCIPLES OF TREATMENT

a. **Tonic neck and labyrinthine reflexes can assist or retard the effects of sensory stimulation**
   - Tonic neck receptors lie in the muscles and skin of the neck region and respond to changes in the relationship of head to the neck.
   - The labyrinthine receptors lie in the ampullae of the semicircular canals and in the vestibule. These receptors are affected by the position of the head in relation to gravity.

b. **Stimulation of specific receptors to produce major reactions**
   The three major reactions that can be produced by stimulation of specific receptors are homeostatic responses via the autonomic nervous system, reflexive protective responses via spinal and brain stem circuits and adaptive responses that require greater integration of all regions of the nervous system.

c. **Four rules of sensory input**
   - A fast brief stimulus produces a large synchronous motor output
   - A fast repetitive sensory input produces a maintained response
   - A maintained sensory input produces a maintained response
   - Slow rhythmical repetitive sensory input deactivates body and mind.

d. **Muscles have different duties**
   Heavy work muscles should be integrated before light work muscles. Primarily refers to the use of upper extremity.

SEQUENCE OF MOTOR DEVELOPMENT

Reciprocal Inhibition (Innervation)

It is an early mobility pattern that sub-serves a protective function. It is a phasic type of movement that requires a contraction of the agonist muscle as the antagonist muscle relaxes.

Cocontraction

It provides stability and is considered to be a tonic pattern. This pattern provides ability to hold a position or an object for longer duration.

Heavy work

Proximal muscles contract and move and the distal segment is fixed.

Skill

It is the highest level of motor control and combines the effort of mobility and stability. To execute a skilled pattern the proximal segment is stabilized while the distal segment moves freely.

ONTOGENIC MOTOR PATTERNS

Supine Withdrawal

It is a total flexion response toward the vertebral level of T 10. This position is protective because the flexion of the neck and the crossing of the arms and leg protects the anterior surface of the body. This position is a mobility posture requiring reciprocal innervations yet it require heavy work of the proximal muscles.

Roll Over

When rolling over the arm and leg flexes on the same side of the body. This movement is a mobility pattern for the extremities and activates the lateral trunk musculature.

Pivot Prone

It demands full range of extension of the neck, shoulders, trunk and lower extremities. It plays an important role in preparation for stability of the extensor muscles in the upright position. It is associated with the labyrinthine righting reaction of the head. The ability to maintain the position indicated integration of the symmetric tonoic labyrinthine (TLR) and tonic neck reflex (TNRs).

Neck Cocontraction

It is the first stability pattern. Cocontraction of neck precedes co-contraction of the trunk and extremities. As the head bobs up and down, the extensors and rotators are stretched to activate flexors and deep neck tonic extensors of the neck. To raise head against gravity the patient needs to have good cocontraction of the flexors and extensors of neck. Neurologically this pattern elicits tonic labyrinthine righting reaction when the face is perpendicular to the floor. As the head flexes it stretches proprioceptors in the neck and upper trapezius, causing them to contract against the forces of gravity. This position also promotes neck stability and extraocular control.

On Elbows

Bearing weight on elbows stretches the trunk musculature to influence the stability of the scapular and glenohumeral regions. It is also inhibitory to symmetric tonic neck reflexes.

All Fours

Follows stability of the neck and shoulders. The lower trunk and lower extremities are brought into a cocontraction pattern. Initially the position is static which develops cocontraction of the trunk flexors and extensors. Eventually, weight shifting forward and backward, side to side and diagonally provides mobility superimposed on the stability phase.

Static Standing

It is thought to be a skill of upper trunk because it frees the upper extremities for prehension and manipulation.

Walking

The gait pattern unites skill mobility and stability. A Normal locomotion entrails the ability to support the body weight, maintain balance and execute the stepping motion. It is a sophisticated process requiring coordinated movement patterns of various parts of the body.

FACILITATION TECHNIQUES

Cutaneous Facilitation

It is used to stimulate the exteroceptors of skin. These receptors respond to the stimuli arising from the external environment. It subserves protective withdrawal responses and produces states of alertness and rapid movements of the limbs.

Light moving touch: Light touch stimuli sends input to limbic structures and increases corticosteroid levels in the blood which helps to increase resistance against diseases, tissue repair and fluid and electrolyte balance. Light moving touch is used to activate superficial mobilizing muscles. These muscles are called as light work group muscles that perform skilled tasks. Neurologically, the light stroke stimulus activates low threshold hair end organs and free nerve endings. The stimuli send impulses along a delta sensory fibers which synapse with the fusimotor system. As a result, light moving touch causes reciprocal innervations, which is clinically seen as phasic withdrawal response. Light moving touch is applied with the fingertip, camel brush or cotton swab.

The frequency of the touch stimulus is three to five strokes with minimum 30 seconds rest in between two strokes. This 30 seconds rest period is important because it prevents presynaptic inhibitory response called primary afferent depolarization which is synaptic mechanism that prevents over stimulation.

Fast brushing: In 1964, Rood introduced a battery-operated brush to stimulate the C fibers which sends many collaterals to the reticular activating system. The stimulation to this system was reported to have its maximal effect 30 minutes after stimulation. Therefore, fast brushing was used before all forms of stimulation because of its prolonged latency effect. Neurologically fast brushing is non-specific high intensity stimulus that increases fusimotor activity of selected muscles. The key to fast brushing is to apply it over the dermatomes of the same segment that supplies the muscles to be facilitated. The stimulus is applied for 3–5 seconds repeated after 30 seconds has elapsed. Fast brushing is contraindicated in the outer ring of the trigeminal nerve where C2 dermatome begins as it has tremendous overlap of free nerve endings, pinna of the ear, along the midline axis of the body.

Icing

Ice is an extreme in thermal facilitation and has been used for facilitation of muscle activity and autonomic nervous system responses. Three uses for icing: It is used for patients who exhibit hypotonia and are in a state of relaxation.

An icing: It probably activates the more myelinated A delta fibers causing reflex withdrawal response in the superficial muscles. The ice is applied to the skin in three quick swipes and the water blotted with terry towel after each swipe. To elicit a withdrawal response of the limbs, the ice is applied to the dorsal web spaces or the palms and soles of hands and feet.

C icing: It is a high intensity nociceptive stimulus that affects the non-specific C fibers. It is used to facilitate postural responses. The ice cube is presses on the skin of a dermatome serving the same spinal segment as the target muscle to be stimulated.

Autonomic icing: It is a stimulus affecting the sympathetic nervous system and probably influences glandular output of thyroid and adrenal glands.

Icing should be avoided in patients with a history of cardiovascular problems.

Proprioceptive facilitatory techniques: It refers to facilitation of muscles spindles, golgi tendon organs, joint receptors and the vestibular apparatus.

a. **Heavy joint compression**: It is defined as joint compression greater than body weight applied through the longitudinal axis of the bone. The amount of force is more than that of body weight above the supporting joint. It is used to facilitate cocontraction of the joint undergoing compression. It can be combined with developmental patterns. The joint compression may be done manually by the therapist or with weighted wrist cuffs and sand bags.
b. **Stretch**: It is a physiologic stimulus used to activate the proprioceptors in selected muscles of the body. Quick stretch employs the principle of reciprocal innervations. The muscle undergoing stretch is facilitated through the Ia afferent of the muscle spindle and by alpha motor neurons.
c. **Intrinsic stretch**: It refers to the use of the intrinsic muscles to promote stability of the scapulohumeral region. In on elbows position, shoulder stability can be enhanced if the patient engages in an activity requiring a resistive grasp. Resistance is a form of stretching because it increases fusimotor activity of the muscle spindle.

   Secondary ending stretch: Roods combined resistance and maintained stretch to facilitate developmental muscle patterns. In principle, anytime a muscle is put on a stretch it fires secondary endings which is always facilitatory to the flexors and inhibitory to the extensors regardless of which muscle is being stretched.
d. **Resistance**: Rood used heavy resistance to stimulate both primary and secondary endings of the muscle spindles. Resistance is used in isotonic

fashion in developmental patterns to influence the stabilizer muscles. In addition, when a muscle contracts against resistance, it assumes a shortened length that causes the muscle spindles to contract, so they readjust to the shorter length.

e. **Tapping**: Tapping over the belly of a muscle with the fingertip. The therapist percusses 3–5 times over the muscle to be facilitated. This may be done during or before the patient is voluntarily contracting. This stimulus acts on the afferents of the muscle spindle and increases the tone of the underlying skeletal muscle.

f. **Vestibular stimulation**: It is a powerful proprioceptive input. The static labyrinthine system can be used to promote extensor patterns of the neck, trunk and extremities. The kinetic labyrinthine system can be used to elicit phasic subcortical responses.

   The vestibular system is stimulated during linear acceleration and deceleration in horizontal and vertical planes and angular acceleration and deceleration.

g. **Therapeutic vibration**: It may be defined as a series of rapid touch stimuli. It has been used for tactile stimulation, to desensitize hypersensitive skin and to produce tonal changes in muscles. vibratory stimuli applied over a muscle belly activate the Ia afferent of the muscle spindle, thereby causing contraction of that muscle, inhibition of the antagonistic muscles and suppression of the stretch reflex. Because vibration is proprioceptory therapeutic modality, it has a short latency period and lasts only as long as the stimulus is applied. To elicit the tonic vibration reflex, the vibrator should be applied over a muscle belly parallel with the muscle fibers.

h. **Osteopressure**: Pressure on bony prominences has been used to facilitate of inhibit voluntary muscle.

INHIBITION TECHNIQUES

Neutral Warmth

It most likely affects the temperature receptors of the hypothalamus and stimulates the parasympathetic nervous system. It can be used for patients with hypertonia (spasticity, rigidity). The procedure entails having a patient assume a recumbent starting position while the entire body is wrapped in a cotton blanket or comforter for approximately 5–10 minutes. It provides a moderate amount of that is homeostatically compatible with the receptors of the hypothalamus.

Gentle Shaking or Rocking

It is a generalized inhibitory technique that uses light joint compression and traction of the cervical vertebrae and slow rhythmic circumduction of the head. This motion affects the proprioceptors of the neck and vestibular apparatus because the joint receptors between the cervical vertebrae and muscle, spindles of the muscles are facilitated. The slow circumduction of the head caused hair cells in the semicircular canals and in the vestibule to alter their rate of discharge.

Slow Stroking

With the patient in prone position, the therapist provides rhythmic, moving deep pressure over the dorsal distribution of the posterior primary rami of the spine. The therapist applies fingertip pressure over the both sides of the spinous processes to affect the nerve ending and sympathetic outflow of the autonomic nervous system. The stroking action is done slowly and continuously from the occiput to the coccyx. The hands are alternated, so that as one hand reaches the bottom of the spine the other hand is starting downwards from the top.

Slow Rolling

The patient is placed in side-lying position the therapist kneels behind the patient and places one hand over rib cage or shoulder and the other hand over the lateral aspect of the patient's pelvis. The patient is rolled slowly from a side lying position to a prone position and back again in a rhythmic fashion.

Light Joint Compression

Joint compression of body weight or less can be used to inhibit spastic muscles around a joint.

Tendinous Pressure

Manual pressure applied to the tendinous insertion of the muscle or across long tendons produces an inhibitory effect. Pressure provided by hard surfaces is preferable to that provide by a soft surfaces.

Maintained Stretch

Rood recommended positioning hypertonic extremities in elongated position for various periods to cause lengthening of the muscle spindles. The rational for this is to reset or bias the afferents of the muscle spindles to a longer position, so that they are less sensitive to stretching.

BIBLIOGRAPHY

1. Pedretti LW, Early MB (Eds). Occupational therapy: Practice skills for physical dysfunction (6th ed). St. Louis, Mosby-Year Book, Inc. 2006.
2. Levitt S. Treatment of cerebral palsy and motor delay (4th ed). Singapore, McGraw-Hill Inc. 2004.
3. Tecklin JS. Pediatric physical therapy (3rd ed). Philadelphia, JB Lippincott Company. 1999.

CHAPTER

6

Motor Relearning Program

Learning Objectives

At the end of the chapter the learner shall be able to:

1. Describe four steps in the execution of the program.
2. Explain seven sections in planning the program.
3. Apply the four steps for each section of the program

INTRODUCTION

Motor relearning program (MRP) is made up of seven sections representing the essential functions of everyday life, most of which are grouped together for ease of reference—upper limb function, orofacial function, motor tasks performed in standing and sitting, standing up and sitting down and walking.

The MRP is commenced as soon as the patient is stable medically. It is intended to be sufficient in its self a program for regaining of control over motor tasks.

The major assumptions are:

- As walking reaching and standing up involves a learning process and that the disabled have the same needs as the non-disabled
- That motor control is exercised in both anticipatory and ongoing modes and that postural adjustments and focal limb movements are interrelated
- Control of specific motor tasks can best be regained by practice of those specific motor tasks and that such tasks need to be practiced in their various environmental contexts
- Sensory input to the motor tasks helps modulate action.

The program assumes the brain's capacity for recovery since it is dynamic and capable of reorganisation and adaptation, and that the functional training may in itself be remedial.

The program is based on four factors known to be essential for the learning of motor skill and therefore assumed to be essential for relearning of motor control following stroke—the elimination of unnecessary muscle activity, feedback, practice and interrelationship between postural adjustment movements.

Throughout the program, emphasis is on the patient consciously practicing particular motor tasks, building-up his awareness of his ability to elicit his muscle activity and control movement, progressing to practice at a more automatic level in order to ensure that the task has been learned and skill therefore acquired.

The four **steps** in motor relearning program are:

Step 1: Analysis of task—observation, comparison, and analysis. Each functional activity is observed in its entirety. Every component of activity is studied in detail taking into consideration the movement taking place at each joint. It is then compared with its normal counterpart. Each activity is then further analyzed in the light of normal activity. The missing components are identified.

Step 2: Practice of missing components—explanations, identification of goal, instruction, practice + verbal and visual feedback + manual guidance. The missing components identified in the first step are practiced. Patient is explained about these components and a goal is identified taking patient into confidence. To achieve this goal, patient is given instruction both verbally and through demonstration. If needed, manual guidance is given to accomplish the goal.

Step 3: Practice of task—explanation, identification of goal, instruction, practice + verbal and feedback + manual guidance, re-evaluation. The missing components are linked together to form a functional activity. This is identified as a goal. It is practiced through the demonstration and verbal feedback. Manual guidance is given wherever needed. It is re-evaluated periodically for improvement in performance.

Step 4: Transference of training—opportunity to practice in context, consistency of practice, organization of self-monitored practice, structured learning environment, involvement of relatives and staff. Once the functional activity is learnt, it is further practiced in context of environment.

Thus, it is only by making a thorough analysis of each task and its associated problems which includes any anatomical, biomechanical physiological and behavioral factors, that the therapist will be able to make correct decisions about intervention. The assumption underlying the analysis is that the observation of motor behavior gives more information about problems of control than the traditional neurological assessments which consists of tests of muscle strength, tone, reflexes and sensations usually performed with the patient in supine and quite unrelated to performance. Furthermore, even if the patient can extend his hip and knee in supine, it does not mean that the patient will be able to activate these muscles appropriately for other tasks such as standing and walking.

The process of analysis continues throughout steps 2 and 3 of the program as therapist continually analyzing and re-evaluating the patients performance and the reasons for success and failure. In order to make decisions about the next stage of treatment or the next instructions to give. This continuous re-evaluation also provides feedback to the therapist about the effectiveness of analysis, decision making and treatment.

Although steps 2 and 3 are separated in order to clarify the part—whole nature of practice, they do in fact overlap. Step 2 only precede step 3 when patient cannot control or contract the necessary muscles and needs to spend some time practicing this component before incorporating it into complex tasks.

There are three important points to be considered in using the program:

1. Motor tasks are practiced in their entirety—many patients in the early stage will be unable to practice the entire activity and will have to practice the components, with emphasis thus on the activation of individual muscle groups.
2. Techniques principally are those associated with and compare the methods of identifying the goal and instructions on how to achieve it, verbal and visual and manual guidance. An explanation and demonstration will help the patient to understand a reason of his difficulty to perform a task that is the necessity of the component on which he has to concentrate on practice.
3. Methods of progression—activities are progressed as soon as the patient has some control. Movements are made more complex by a decrease in the manual guidance and feedback, by alterations in speed and by adding variety. As the patient regains some skill in the activity, he

should be exposed to different environmental conditions in order to improve his performance and to enable him to develop the flexibility required for performance in an open environment.

Seven sections of MRP represent the basic functional activities considered imperative for activities of daily living. They are described below:

UPPER LIMB DYSFUNCTION

Most daily activities involve complex movements of the upper limbs. Motor tasks performed by the upper limb thus illustrates very well the two fundamental problems in motor control—the degrees of freedom and the problem of context specific or content conditioned variability. In daily life, thc goal of the arm is often the placement of hand.

There are certain prerequisites for effective use of the upper limb.

These are, 1. The ability to seed what one is doing; 2. The ability to make postural adjustments which occur with arm movement and which free the hands for manipulation; and 3. Sensory information.

The major function of the arm is to enable the hand to be positioned in space for manipulation. Hence, the essential components involved in reaching are shoulder abduction, forward flexion, extension and elbow flexion and extension. The major function of the hand is to grasp, release and manipulate objects for specific purposes. Hence, the essential components are: Radial deviation combined with wrist extension, wrist flexion and extension holding an object, palmar abduction and rotation at the carpometacarpal (CMC) joint of the thumb flexion and conjunct rotation of the metacarpophalangeal (MCP) joints of the individual joints with the IP joints in some flexion supination and pronation of the forearm while holding an object.

Step 1: Analysis of Tasks

Common Problems and Compensatory Strategies

Arm: Poor scapular movement (particulary lateral rotation and protraction) and persistent depression of the shoulder.

Hand: Difficulty grasping with wrist in extension in the absence of wrist extensor activity, the long finger flexors act to flex the wrist and fingers. Difficulty in flexing and extending the MCP joints with IP joints in some flexion in order to position the fingers while grasping and releasing an object.

In addition, following are the common sequel to the stroke, all of which are probably preventable. Habitual posturing of the limb leading to length associated changes in the soft tissues of the shoulder, wrist, thumb and fingers, compensation with intact arm, use of intact arm to move the affected limb learned non-use of the affected arm.

Analysis of the painful shoulder: Soft tissue injury with resultant pain, stiffness and subluxation will usually result from four mechanical factors pinching of the soft tissues against the acromion, friction of the soft tissues against the bone, traction to soft tissues and soft tissue contracture.

If pain alone is a problem treatment may include peripheral joint mobilization, interferential and transcutaneous nerve stimulation. If chronic inflammation exists heat or ultrasound may stimulate a normal repair process. there are two possible components of joint stiffness—adaptive tissue contracture secondary to disuse and adhesions between normally free sliding structures.

Steps 2 and 3: Practice of Upper Limb Function

Motor activity can usually be elicited early with the patient in supine with his arm in elevation. Also a muscle may be activated as part of one particular synergy before it can be activated as a part of another.

Following points should be kept in mind—arm movements that must be trained early following stroke. Hand movements must not be left until there is some recovery of function around shoulder. As soon as isolated muscle action is elicited, this must be practiced and extended into meaningful tasks, with the patient gaining control over increasing ranges of movement.

All muscle activity unnecessary to movement being attempted must be eliminated consciously by the patient.

Gross therapist controlled patterns of movement of the upper limbs should be avoided as these will not allow either the therapist or the patient to be aware of any minimal muscle activity present and they will tend to encourage only active muscles.

Activity should be elicited first in the position of greatest advantage to the muscle. It is important that in due course of time the manual guidance required when there is insufficient muscle activity is changed to a verbal guidance.

If a muscle does not contract in a particular set of conditions vary the conditions.

The patient should not be encouraged to practice movements which are not functionally significant.

The therapist should not think in terms of strengthening the muscles in general sense. The objective is to help the patient elicit muscle activity and to train him to control this activity for specific tasks. As he practices various tasks, he will acquire the appropriate muscular strength and endurance relatively easily provided. He is given the opportunity to work to the point of muscular fatigue.

Tasks involving both arms should be encouraged as early as possible. In certain tasks the two limbs seems to function as part of one synergy which includes the objects being manipulated and because of the apparently context specific nature of the control processes, these tasks will need to be specifically practiced to be relearned.

Step 4: Transference of Training into Daily Life

If the patient is to achieve his potential recovery of upper limb function there are four points which must be considered.

1. He must not suffer secondary soft tissue injury—for this patient should not be encouraged to move the affected limb passively and he should not be given pulley exercises. Both activities fail to take into account the normal scapulohumeral rhythm and therefore increase the likelihood of soft tissue injury in the shoulder region.
2. He must not be allowed or encouraged to develop non-learned use of his affected arm, by performing activities that involve movement of the affected limb by the intact limb or by moving, using the intact limbs.
3. During the day patient should practice particular components or movements on which the therapist considers he should concentrate. Movements which are too difficult to practice on his own can be practiced mentally.
4. Persistent posturing of the limb is a particular problem in the early stages following stroke. The flaccid or inactive limb is held by the side in internal rotation and flexion, causing length associated changes to occur, probably quite rapidly and allowing the glenohumeral joint to sublux downwards.

OROFACIAL FUNCTIONS

It comprises of various activities, such as swallowing, facial expression, ventilation and motor aspects of speech production. Following stroke all these activities are affected interfering with eating, communication and socialization.

In the first few days, it is the inefficient swallowing which causes the greatest dysfunction. The resultant drooling, aspiration and difficulty ingesting the food bring about a poor nutritional state.

It is particularly important that normal swallowing is retrained as early as possible.

Swallowing is a highly complex and integrated neuromuscular task. The essential components are—jaw closure, lip closure, elevation of the posterior third of the tongue to close off posterior oral cavity, elevation of lateral borders of tongue.

There are certain prerequisites which are necessary for effective swallowing: Sitting position, control of breathing in relation to swallowing, normal reflex activity.

Analysis of orofacial function involves—observation of the alignment and movements of lips, jaws and tongue, intraoral digital examination of tongue and cheeks, observation of eating and drinking, difficulty with swallowing, lack of control over orofacial musculature, in particular. open jaw, poor lip seal, immobile tongue.

This will result in—drooling, food collecting between cheeks and gums. Although this is often attributed to lack of muscle activity in the cheek, a major factor is probability the immobility of tongue. Altered threshold to stimulation will result in diminished awareness, hypersensitivity.

Imbalance of facial movements and expression—this is the result of lack of motor control of the lower part of the face on the affected side, together with over activity and unopposed activity of the face on the intact side.

Lack of emotional control—this lack of control is demonstrated by the outbursts of uncontrolled crying which the patient has difficulty in modifying or stopping. Poor breathing control—because of poor control over the soft palate or motor incompetency demonstrated by a difficulty to take a deep breath holding a breath or and controlling a prolonged expiration thus making communication difficult.

Steps 2 and 3

The most efficient position for swallowing and therefore eating is sitting patient should be sitting way back in chair with his neck and trunk erect.

Intraoral techniques should be interrupted frequently and jaw held closed in order to allow the patient to swallow. Presence of saliva and closure of jaw and lips will combine with the improved muscular activity of the tongue to trigger off swallowing.

Step 4: Transference of Treatment into Daily Life

During all training sessions, the therapist monitors the patient's facial posture while he concentrates on various tasks, indicating him when his jaw is open and reminding him to keep his mouth closed.

SITTING UP OVER THE SIDE OF BED

Most people when they sit up over the side of the bed, go from supine to sitting up, use the hands to leverage and swing the legs over the side of the bed. In the early stages of stroke, it is practical and more effective for the patient to be assisted to turn onto his intact side and sit up from this position. There are three reasons for this—it avoids unrestrained use of the intact arm which results when the patient pulls himself up from supine to sitting, it is a quick and easy way for the patient to sit up with minimal help from another person and it gives him the idea as to how to do it himself.

Essential components—turning on the side-rotation and flexion of the neck, hip and knee flexion, flexion of shoulder and protraction of the shoulder girdle rotation within the trunk.

Sitting up over the side of the bed—lateral flexion of the neck, lateral flexion of trunk, legs lifted and lowered over the side of the bed.

Step 1: Analysis of the Sitting up Over the Side of the Bed

In turning to the intact side, the patient may demonstrate particular difficulty in—flexion of the hip and knee on the affected side, flexion of the shoulder and protraction of the shoulder girdle. These problems will result in—appropriate compensatory movements on the intact side also failure to make an attempt to move affected arm passively across his body may indicate that he is neglecting the affected side.

In sitting up over the side of the bed, the following problems may occur in compensation for the depressed muscle activity—patient rotates neck and flexes it forward instead of laterally. This usually occurs because of poor lateral trunk movement. Patient pulls with intact hand instead of laterally flexing the neck and trunk. Patient hooks intact leg under affected leg in order to get legs over the side of the bed. This will shift his weight back as he attempts to sit up.

Step 2 and 3: Practice of Missing Components

Therapist assists on the intact side. It is important that he does not have to struggle. The therapist encourages him to turn his head, assists him to bring his shoulder and arm forward, and to flex his hips and knees. She may have to adjust his pelvis and legs in order to provide a stable base of support once he has turned on to his side.

Step 4: Transference of Training into Daily Life

The patient should not spend any more time in the bed than is necessary for medical reasons, nor should he spend any more time lying down than is necessary for sleeping or for retraining of upper limb function in therapy sessions. The lying position reinforces drowsiness, confusion and feelings of helplessness and provokes the symptoms of deprivation. Early assumption of the erect position has a stimulating effect on the CNS, counteracts depression, enables the patient to gain control over the bladder function and oral function, gives relevant visual input and encourages communication. The sitting position appears to aid in emptying the bladder and bowel. If the patient must remain in bed, the task of getting onto a bed pan is made easier if the nurse flexes his affected hip and knee, hold the foot firmly onto the bed and ask him to flex his intact hip and knee, push down through his heels and lift his buttocks. This should not be attempted with more than one pillow under the head as flexion of the neck makes it extend the hips.

BALANCED SITTING

The ability to achieve sitting position requires that the body alignment be appropriate to each task and that the correct preparatory and ongoing postural adjustments can be made as shifts in center of gravity (COG) occur throughout performance of the task. balanced sitting is defined as ability to sit without using undue muscle activity to move about in sitting, to perform a wide variety of motor tasks and to move in and out of the sitting position.

Essential components: Body alignment in sitting depends on number of factors—1. What one is sitting on, 2. What one is doing, 3. General body posture.

The following essentials of sitting alignment related to sitting up straight. Feet and knees close together, weight evenly distributed, flexion of the hips with extension of the trunk, head balanced on level surfaces, the ability to make preparatory postural adjustments and ongoing postural adjustments, which are specific to the movement of motor tasks being performed.

Step 1: Analysis of Balanced Sitting

Consists of observation of the patient's alignment in quite sitting, analysis of his ability to adjust self-initiated movement of the limbs, trunk, and head as he performs the graded variety of motor tasks. The therapist notes his behavior, including extraneous movements and compensatory strategies.

Common compensatory strategies—wide base of support voluntary restriction of movement. Patient shuffles feet instead of making adjustments with appropriate body segments. Protective support on hand or arm or grabbing for support with minimal movement. Patient leans forwards and backwards when the task requires that the body weight should be shifted sideways.

Steps 2 and 3: Practice of Missing Components

During the first few sessions, if the patients balance in sitting is poor, he should sit on a low firm stool with his feet on the floor. As he progresses in his ability to move around, he should also practice various tasks while sitting on various types of seat. As the patient practices moving about the therapist ensures that he makes necessary adjustments and does not shuffle his feet, widen his base or wriggle around.

Step 4: Transference of Training into Daily Life

Emphasis in this step is on organizing the resting posture of the flaccid arm to be varied throughout the day and the patient to have the opportunity to practice standing up. The patient should remember to shift his body weight from one buttock to another frequently passively. Throughout the day, patient is sitting on a chair which is, he should sit on a chair from which it is possible to stand up.

STANDING UP AND SITTING DOWN

Description of normal function: In standing up one or both feet move backwards this gives base under the COG as it is moved forward. Inclination of the extended trunk forward at the hips with forward movement of the knees brings the COG over the feet and enables the weight of the body to be shifted forwards and upwards. If the chair prevents the feet from far moving backwards, the trunk has to move forward or one has to come to the edge of chair.

In sitting down, one probably looks at the where abouts of the chair by turning to look, feeling for the chair with the hand or feeling it against the back of the leg. The hips and knees flex, the trunk is inclining forward, so that the COG can be shifted backwards. The body weight is lowered to the chair by a lengthening or eccentric contraction of the extensors. It is the forward inclination of trunk caused by flexion of hips and the forward movement of the knees which enable the pelvis to move backwards and downwards towards the chair.

Essential components:

- Standing up—foot placement, inclination of the trunk forward by flexion of hips with extended neck and spine, movement of the knees backwards, extension of hips and knees for final standing alignment.
- Sitting down: Inclination of the trunk forward by flexion of hips with extended neck and spine, movement of the knees forward and knee flexion.

Step 1: Analysis of Standing and Sitting Down

The stroke patient, because of his lack of force generating capacity of the affected leg, is compelled to shift his weight on the intact leg when he attempts to stand up and sit down and soon this become a learned compensatory strategy.

The common problems are as follows—weight is borne principally through the intact side, inability to shift COG sufficiently forwards, i.e. inability to move shoulders forward over the feet and move knees forwards. Patient rises to shift forward by flexing the trunk and head instead of hips or by wriggling to the edge of chair. Failure to place the affected foot makes the patient to stand up and sit down with all weight taken through the intact leg.

Step 2: Practice of Missing Components

To train trunk inclination forward at hips.

Step 3: Practice of Standing up and Sitting Down

If the patient is very weak, overweight or unable to generate sufficient force to stand up, he may need two people to assist him to stand up. Practice of standing up may be facilitated by a higher chair which eliminates some of the difficulty involved in generating the force patients who have difficulty in standing up may find it easier to gain some muscle control as they sit down, and practice of sitting down may actually help them improve control over the more difficult action of standing up.

Step 4: Transference of Training into Daily Life

There is a great improvement in morale and lifestyle of the patient when he can stand up from the chair on his own. The patient has to be able to stand up and sit down by himself in order to change from one chair to another, to go to the toilet and to practice walking. To become efficient in this task he needs the opportunity to practice on his own. This will require the therapist organizes a written checklist of what he is to practice and what specific he is to achieve. It is proved that the standing up from a higher chair reduces the stress on hips and knees. The joint moments needed are significantly reduced indicating that the less muscle activity is reduced. Members of staff and relatives need to understand the basic principle involved, how to assist, how to reinforce and monitor the performance. Particularly in this task there is a tendency for the patient to practice standing up one way while with the therapist in the physiotherapy area and for him to stand up in a different way in another environments or on his own. Some training sessions with the therapist in these environments may help overcome the problem.

Usually there is no consistency in the Program because patient may practice in one way in therapy sessions and another way throughout the day. The therapist should know that what he practices is what he will learn.

BALANCED STANDING

It involves the ability to stand relatively still without using undue muscular activity, to move about in standing to perform a wide variety of tasks, to move in and out of standing position and to take steps. Standing is not a static posture but involves a constant slight movement called postural sway. Even small shift of gravity involves some preparatory and ongoing muscular activity.

Body alignment is more critical in standing than in sitting since the base of support is small. A well aligned position requires less energy than a poorly aligned position. Body alignment in standing depends on number of factors—what one is standing on, what one is doing, one's general posture and other factors such as age and sex. Essentials of standing alignment—feet few inches apart, hips in front of ankles, shoulders over hips, head balanced on level shoulders, erect trunk.

Essential components of balanced standing—preparatory postural adjustments and ongoing postural adjustments which are specific to the goals of either standing still or performing particular motor tasks.

Step 1: Analysis of Balanced Standing

Consists of observation of patient's alignment in quite standing, analysis of his ability to make adjustments to the self-initiated movements of the limbs trunk and head as he performs a graded variety of motor tasks. Common compensatory strategies-wide base of support, voluntary restriction of movements, patient shuffles instead of walking, patient takes as step prematurely. Patient flexes hips instead of dorsiflexing at ankles in reaching forward and moves at trunk instead of hips and feet when reaching sideways, use of arms for grabbing.

Step 2 and 3: Practice of Balanced Standing

All stroke patients when they first attempt to stand are off balance. Many of them tend to drift to one side or fall backwards. Many patients react by shifting most of their weight on intact side. From the start, patient should be informed as to what is going wrong and how to correct it. He should be explained that the solution does not lie in holding on with his hands but in gaining control over his pelvis legs, and trunk. Similarly, the therapist should not panic and react by holding him up. If she resists the impulse and gives him a strategy for overcoming the problem, he will quickly learn to make an effective adjustment.

It is important that the patient stands within the first few days and with weight through both legs. This enables him to commence training in balancing and walking skills. A rapid regaining of balance increases awareness of bilaterality, and position in space and of body parts which is particularly important for people with unilateral spatial neglect or diminished kinesthetic sensation. Standing prevents contracture of, particularly of calf muscles and the hip flexor muscles, provides motivation and encouragement and as balance improves, self-confidence in early stages it increases the level of alertness and probably influences bladder control. Standing with weight through the affected leg in correct alignment may be one of the factors in minimizing the development of spasticity in the leg.

Some patients due to unilateral spatial neglect or inability to contract their leg muscles will find it easier to stand if the knee is controlled in a splint. Practice of balanced sitting should not be expected to transfer into bilateral standing. It is also probable that, following a stroke, a person will not automatically regain the ability to move about in standing with necessary postural adjustments without specific training in standing. Hence, to postpone standing because the person has no balance makes little sense.

Step 4: Transference of Training into Daily Living

The patient should be helped to stand up and should begin training in standing from his first therapy session if his medical condition is satisfactory. He should also have the opportunity to practice during the day. He should know to stand with his body segments aligned correctly and with weight borne through the affected leg. He should be given written instructions of the major points, so that he can monitor his own performance.

It should be noted that the patient has to be able to stand up and sit down in order to practice standing and walking. He may need assistance to stand up or the therapist may need arrange for him to have a chair of suitable height and firmness from which he is able to stand up.

The patient should spend short periods during the day standing at a table. Lack of practice of standing with hips forward results in shortening of the calf muscles which will prevent him from standing with weight through the affected leg and will also interfere significantly with walking training.

WALKING

Bipedal level walking is a very unstable movement. perturbations result from the large gravitational and forward momentum forces acting while the body is supported on one limb for 80% of the time. This is inherently unstable and requires complex control.

Step 1: Analysis of walking-stance phase of Affected leg

- Lack of extension of hip and dorsiflexion of ankles
- Lack of controlled knee flexion- extension from 15°
- Excessive lateral horizontal shift of pelvis
- Excessive downward pelvic tilt on the intact side associated with excessive pelvic shift to the affected side.

Swing phase of the affected leg:

- Lack of knee flexion at toe off.
- Lack of hip flexion
- Lack of knee extension plus ankle dorsiflexion on heel strike.

In addition, the patient lacks the idea of sequencing of components and of the rhythm and timing of walking.

- Analysis and subsequent training of walking always begin with the affected leg in stance phase—it is essential that the patient acquire the ability to bear weight through his leg in normal alignment with hip extension, controlled knee extension and ability to shift the COG approximately 2.5 cm laterally to the affected side. The patients will then be able to practice stepping forward with his intact leg and this will position his affected leg for swing phase.
- Difficulty translating or shifting the COG laterally—in order to free the intact leg for swinging forward. Many a times patient shifts their pelvis too far laterally. This results in a compensatory tilt of the pelvis downwards on the intact side. ipsilateral hip abduction contractions and contralateral trunk side flexors causes this too far lateral shift of the pelvis. Lack of active terminal knee extension or locked position of knee joint will affect the normal tibiofemoral angle, which in turn will affect degree of lateral pelvic shift. He is also associated with lack of hip extension which not only disturbs the normal body alignment but also affects the mechanism which controls the excessive lateral pelvic shift.

- Inability to extend the affected hip—which in turn results in inability to shift the COG forward when the step is taken forward. This results in inability to move the body forward until the unaffected foot is on the ground and excessive extension of the unaffected side takes place with the affected side hip in flexed position. The patient flexes his trunk when the step is taken with the affected leg as a result of lack of hip extension and immediately takes a short step with unaffected side.
- Lack of knee control throughout the stance phase—initially, it results in buckling of the knee as soon as the patient takes weight on the affected side. Later, a patient learns to lock it in hyperextension until the complete stance phase on affected side is over. Thus, knee is not allowed to be flexed prior to swing phase. This is because of lack of knee control especially in 0–15° extension. This further results in compensatory short calf muscles which prevents hip extension and hence ability of the body to shift the COG forward in order to keep moving forward. If the patient has some activity in the quadriceps he is able to maintain some amount of knee flexion at mid stance.
- Lack of knee flexion at toe off—in a normal gait, knee flexion occurs at the end of stance phase when the extremity prepares itself for swing phase, when the hip is in extension. in patients with stroke, this knee flexion is not present. this produces compensation in abnormal swing forward of the affected leg may be in the form of hitching the leg up or abduction of the hip or backward tilting of the pelvis.
- Lack of active dorsiflexion at the end of stance phase—this result in inability to clear the ground and the foot is dragged if no compensatory mechanism is adapted by patient. The compensatory mechanisms can be in the form of hitching the pelvis up or abduction of hip to shorten the extremity.
- A wide base of support while walking—this is due to poor balance and fear of fall. It is also because of inability of the patient to control the affected leg during the swing phase. This may result in keeping the affected extremity in too much abducted position. In addition, instance phase, the poor alignment which results from lack of hip extension and excessive lateral horizontal shift towards the affected side may result in intact foot stepping out to the side.

Step 2: Practice of Missing Components

Aims are to train hip extension throughout the stance phase, to train knee control in stance phase, to train lateral horizontal pelvic shift, to train flexion of the knee at the start of swing phase and to train knee extension and foot dorsiflexion at heel strike.

For this, the patient is taken in the appropriate position instructions are given to maintain proper alignment of the body and then with demonstration or verbal feedback the patient is taught to activate the needed muscles at the given time during gait.

Step 3: Practice of Walking

Practice of individual components of walking should be followed by practice of walking itself which enables the patient to put these components together in their proper sequence. To begin with the patient steps with his intact leg first. With realignment of the body in preparation for the next step, patient takes a next step with affected side.

His new abilities now need to be stretched to their limits with increasing further complexity of walking. This can be done by practicing with stepping over the objects of different heights, walking combined with other activities, varying the speed of walking.

Step 4: Transference of Training into Daily Life

When the treatment session is over the patient can set himself a goal of how much he walks on the first day and can extend the distance and/or time taken on the next day. The patient needs the opportunity to practice himself or with other members of staff or relatives. He is given written instructions, so he knows what he should concentrate on. Standing or walking aids such as parallel bars or a three point cane will alleviate only transiently the patient's balance problems and when used continually will worsen the problems since control mechanisms rapidly adapt to the additional feedback and support provided.

BIBLIOGRAPHY

1. Carr JH, Shepherd RB. A motor relearning Program. London: William Heinmann. 1987.
2. Dickstein R, Hochermann S, Pillar T, Shaham R. Stroke Rehabilitation. Three exercise Therapy approaches. Phys Ther. 1986;66:1233-8.

CHAPTER

7

Myofascial Release

Learning Objectives

At the end of the chapter the learner shall be able to:

1. Describe the principle
2. Describe the mechanism of action
3. Describe the basic technique of application
4. Explain effects of MFR

Myofascial release is a form of soft tissue therapy used to treat somatic dysfunction and accompanying pain and restriction of motion. This is accomplished by relaxing contracted muscles, increasing circulation, increasing venous and lymphatic drainage, and stimulating the stretch reflex of muscles and overlying fascia. It differs from other stretching techniques. It relies mainly on the feedback received by the therapist from the patient nonverbally through the patient's tissues. It is the therapist who determines how much, how long and how forceful stretching will be, according to the response of the patient's body. By utilizing the feedback received from the patient's body, the therapist can effectively stretch restricted structures in the manner comfortable to the patient than can be done with traditional stretching techniques, this can be done without sacrificing the effectiveness of the stretch. It is a very safe technique and there is no danger that the therapist will inadvertently overstretch the soft tissues of the body when the techniques are being applied correctly.

General guidelines: First the area to be stretched is palpated to determine the area of restriction. Next the tissues are stretched gently along the direction of line of muscle fibers until a resistance to further stretch is felt. This stretch position is held until the soft tissues are felt to relax. The relaxation is due to the dissipation of a restriction and is called a release. It is sensed by the therapist and patient as softening or let go. Then the tissues are stretched further to take up the slack created by the release and are held in a new elongated position. The process is repeated until the tissues are in a fully elongated position or until no further stretching can be tolerated.

Any muscle that allows the placement of two hands or even two fingers can be gently stretched to relieve myofascial restrictions. Hand placement should be comfortable for both patient and therapist. For large muscle groups such as the erector spinae, the middle trapezii or the quadriceps femoris one may gain better leverage by crossing the hands. For small muscles like the masseter only one or two fingers are needed without crossing the hands. A hand of finger is placed on the proximal to the attachments of the muscles to be stretched, using just enough pressure to stretch the superficial skin and fascia and to stretch the underlying muscles in the direction of muscle fibers. This needs to be done in a firm manner. This position is held until all the soft tissues are felt to relax, then it is stretched again, taking up the additional slack created by the release. This process is repeated until no further stretch is possible and both the muscles and related soft tissues are in a fully elongated position. Slowly and gently the stretch pressure is released and restrictions are re-evaluated.

TECHNIQUES FOR MYOFASCIAL RELEASE THERAPY

The main approach of every technique is more or less similar. A physical therapist locates the restricted fascia portion and applies light stretch to the area. Pressure application is repeated for several times, until the restricted fascia can be stretched properly. The same procedure is followed for the treatment of other sore and restricted spots. Based on the therapy approach, there are two myofascial release techniques, namely direct and indirect therapy.

Direct Release: According to this technique, the functionality of the restricted fascia is improved by using low force directly on the affected spots. For stretching the trigger points, the physical therapist may apply pressure of a few kilogram by using elbows, forearm, knuckles or other therapy tools. This direct technique involves the manipulation of deep tissues by pressure application. Under this method, the physician first locates the barrier within the soft tissue, holds it with pressure for 50–60 seconds and release it gently. As per the patient's medical problem, direct release may be conducted on the face, head, neck, trunk, cervical portion, pelvis, thigh and feet.

Indirect Release: In this technique, a very low pressure of about a few grams is applied to the fascia. The objective of this method is to increase the heat and blood circulation in the restricted fascia. Following this, the body's natural ability allows the fascia to relax and stretch on its own. For performing the indirect technique, the therapist uses fingers to lightly press on the restricted fascia for about 4 minutes, after which the pressure is released slowly. This way, the built up of muscle tension is balanced. Very often, therapeutic pulse is observed during the procedure of indirect therapy.

In recent times, physical therapist conduct these techniques by using fitness accessories like foam rollers, flexible bags and therapy balls. Overall, myofascial release therapy is a gentle and safe procedure for body relaxation. As more people are engaged into this therapy, certain self-performing techniques are suggested to carry out at home. However, prior to doing any self-techniques, one should always consult a therapist regarding the positions, activities and their effects.

To further improve the effect of myofascial release, prolonged corrective positioning with use of postural wedges or therapeutic balls or both, to sustain appropriate pressure to release fascia over time. Also , once fascia is released , it is important to exercise muscles to strengthen resistance to the fascia tightening up once again in gravity.

Effects of MFR

- **Relaxation of contracted muscles and soft tissues:** The MFR has a direct effect on the contracted soft tissues. By positioning and movement of the hands of therapist along the direction of muscle fibers, there is a release of the tightness .
- **Increases circulation:** Because of the tightness, the intermuscular space is reduced thereby compromising on the vascular supply. Release of the tightened structures helps to regain the circulation thereby nourishing the muscles and soft tissues. This further results in removal of metabolites from the affected area, thus causing pain relief associated with tightness.

- **Increasing venous and lymphatic drainage:** With MFR efficiency of the muscles to contract and relax is improved. This results in better pumping out of the extracellular fluid , thus improving lymphatic drainage. Venous return is improved owing to the effective pumping action of the muscles.
- **Stimulation of the stretch reflex:** Considering the altered nervous system in patients with neuromuscular diseases, MFR causes stimulation of stretch reflex. The extremity or the part to be treated is stretched to its physiological limit in order to overcome the tightness. This results in stimulation of the golgi tendon organs situated inside the muscles which in turn causes stimulation of stretch reflex. This is helpful to elicit a voluntary contraction in completely flaccid muscles.

Practical application: When there is a neuromuscular disease that is present along with hypertonicity in the muscles, MFR can be used effectively to reduce tone in the muscles. It works on the principles of reflex inhibition because of static positioning. In patients with neuromuscular diseases there is a superimposed musculoskeletal dysfunction. This might be in the form of tightened soft tissues specially the muscles because of which the ability of a muscle to function is hampered. This results in functional restriction even in the absence of any direct pathology in musculoskeletal structures. Because of continuous posturing in one position or in a wrong position, these patients develops contractures in muscles and other soft tissues.

Following are Some of the Examples of MFR Techniques

Releases in the shoulder and arm region can be given by using the technique called Arm Pull. In this, with the subject in supine lying position, therapist holds the patients hand one on thenar side and other on hypothenar side. During the arm pull, interossoeous muscle and palmar fascia is stretched at the same time. Then the therapist stands in such a way towards the foot end of the patient as if to apply longitudinal traction to whole of the upper extremity. Gentle traction is applied to whole of the extremity. It is released as soon as the therapist feels relaxation of the soft tissues. Again traction is applied and process is repeated twice or thrice.

MFR to pectoral muscles: Upper fibers of pectoralis can be stretched by placing both hands on the muscle in a crossed manner. The therapist is standing at head end of the patient facing towards the feet. The shoulder is abducted to 45°. The hands are then moved medially and laterally across the horizontal fibers. Similarly the lower fibers which fan from the ribs and sternum should also be stretched. Pectoralis muscle can also be stretched by use of arm pull technique, angling the arm along the direction of muscle fibers.

Erector spinae muscle can also be stretched in prone position with arms crossed and moving in a cephalad and caudal direction.

BIBLIOGRAPHY

1. DiGiovnna. E Schiowitz S, Dowling D J. Myofascial (soft tissue) Techniques (Chapter 12). An osteopathic approach to diagnosis and treatment. 3rd edn. Philadelphia, PA: Lippincott Williams and Wilkins 1991.
2. Manheim CF. Myofascial release manual (4th edn.) Thorofare, New Jersey: Slack 1990.
3. Stanborough M. Direct release myofascial technique: an illustrated guide for practitioners. Edinburgh: Churchill Livingstone 2004.

CHAPTER

8

Proprioceptive Neuromuscular Facilitation

Learning Objectives

At the end of the chapter the learner shall be able to:

1. Define PNF
2. Describe principles of PNF
3. Describe mass movement patterns in detail
4. Describe techniques of emphasis of PNF

INTRODUCTION

Techniques of PNF are methods of placing specific demands in order to secure a desired response.

Facilitation by definition means the promotion or hastening of any natural process, the reverse of inhibition, specifically the effect produced in nerve tissue by the passage of an impulse. The resistance of the nerve tissue is diminished so that a second application of the stimulus evokes the reaction more easily.

Proprioceptive means receiving stimulation within the tissues of the body.

Neuromuscular means pertaining to the nerves and muscles.

Therefore, techniques of PNF are defined as methods of promoting or hastening the response of the neuromuscular mechanism through stimulation of the proprioceptors.

The normal neuromuscular system becomes integrated and efficient without awareness of individual muscle action, reflex activity and a multiple of other neurophysiological reactions. The deficient neuromuscular system is inadequate to meet the demands of life, in proportion to the degree of deficiency. Response may be limited as a result of faulty development, trauma or diseases of nervous system or the musculoskeletal system. Deficiencies present themselves in terms of limitation of movement as evidenced by weakness, incoordination, adaptive shortening or immobility of joints muscle spasm or spasticity.

PRINCIPLES OF PNF

Patterns of Motion

The patterns of motion for PNF are mass movement patterns and are basic to all other techniques. Mass movement is a characteristic of normal motor activity and is in keeping with Beevor's axiom that the brain knows nothing of individual muscle action but knows only of movement. It is a means of placing specific demands on the muscles that must be in specific combinations of motions which are optimum for the specific sequence of muscles primarily responsible for the movement, and it must allow these muscles to contribute their components of action consistently.

The mass movement patterns are spiral and diagonal in character. This is in keeping with the spiral and rotatory characteristics of the skeletal system of bones and joints and the ligamentous structures.

There are two diagonals of motion for each of the major parts of the body. Each diagonal is made up of two patterns which are antagonistics to each other's. Each pattern has a major component of flexion or extension, there being two flexion and two extension patterns for each of the major parts, these major components are always combined with two other components.

Motion Components

Each spiral and diagonal pattern is a 3 component motion with respect to all of the joints or pivots of action participating in movement. The three components include flexion or extension, abduction or adduction and rotation.

Major Muscle Components

The major muscle components of a given pattern are related by their topographical alignment upon the skeletal system and are primarily responsible for the movement. The muscles secondarily responsible for a pattern are those muscles which are most closely related by location and function.

Line of Movement

The spiral and diagonal patterns of facilitation provide for an optimal contraction of the major muscle components. A pattern of motion that is optimal for a specific action of muscles to contract from their completely lengthened state to their completely shortened state, when the pattern is performed through the full ROM.

Cooperative functions of muscles since 3 components are considered with reference to all joints or pivots participating in a pattern, the major muscle components cooperatively contribute to the 3 components as far as their topographical location and structure will permit. The function of an individual muscle action is a 3 component action. The motion component which places the most stretch on a muscle determines its primary action component.

Mass Movement Patterns

Neck

- Flexion with rotation to the right
- Extension with rotation to the left
- Rotation to the left

Upper trunk

- Flexion with rotation to the right
- Extension with rotation to the left
- Rotation to the left

Lower trunk

- Flexion with rotation to the left
- Extension with rotation to the right

Table 8.1: Upper Extremity D1 pattern

Joint	Flexion	Extension
Scapula	Elevation, abduction, rotation	Depression, adduction, rotation
Shoulder	Flexion, adduction external rotation	Extension, abduction internal rotation
Elbow	Flexion or extension	Flexion or extension
Forearm	Supination	Pronation
Wrist and hand	Flexion to the radial side, finger flexion and adduction, thumb adduction	Extension to the ulnar side, finger extension and abduction, thumb in palmar abduction

Table 8.2: Upper Extremity D2 pattern

Joint	Flexion	Extension
Scapula	Elevation, adduction, rotation	Depression, abduction, rotation
Shoulder	Flexion, abduction External rotation	Extension, adduction internal rotation
Elbow	Flexion or extension	Flexion or extension
Forearm	Supination	Pronation
Wrist and Hand	Extension to the radial side, finger extension and abduction, thumb extension	Flexion to the ulnar side, finger flexion and adduction, thumb in opposition

Table 8.3: Lower Extremity D1 pattern

Joint	Flexion	Extension
Hip	Flexion Abduction External rotation	Extension Adduction Internal rotation
Knee	Flexion/extension	Flexion/extension
Ankle and Foot	Dorsiflexion inversion	Plantarflexion eversion
Toe	Extension	Flexion

Table 8.4: Lower Extremity D2 pattern

Joint	Flexion	Extension
Hip	Flexion Abduction External rotation	Extension Adduction Internal rotation
Knee	Flexion/extension	Flexion/extension
Ankle and Foot	Dorsiflexion Inversion	Plantarflexion Inversion
Toe	Extension	Flexion

Neck, Upper Trunk and Lower Trunk

The patterns of neck and upper trunk are described as flexion or extension with rotation to the right or left. The neck patterns are key to the upper trunk patterns and the components of a specific neck pattern are continued in the homologous pattern of the upper trunk. The lower trunk patterns are described as flexion or extension with rotation to the right or left. The bilateral asymmetrical lower extremity patterns are the key to lower trunk patterns and contribute their repetitive components of motion. The distal parts of the extremities move across the midline of the trunk. Motions of the pelvis include elevation of the pelvic brim as the counterpart of extension, and rotation to the right or left.

Upper and Lower Extremities

Proximal pivots: Motions named according to the motion occurring at proximal joints. In the upper extremity shoulder flexion and extension are combined with abduction and adduction. External rotation is consistent with flexion and internal rotation with extension. In the lower extremity, hip flexion and extension are combined with abduction and adduction and with external and internal rotation. Adduction is consistent with external rotation and abduction is consistent with internal rotation.

Intermediate pivots, i.e. knee and elbow may remain straight or flexed. The rotation and gliding motion of these joints are consistently in line with the rotation and abduction or adduction of hip or shoulder.

Distal pivots: They are consistent with proximal components. In the upper extremity supination of forearm and motion of wrist towards the radial side are consistent with flexion and external rotation of shoulder. In the lower extremity, plantarflexion of ankle and foot are consistent with hip extension and dorsiflexion are consistent with hip flexion. Inversion of foot motion towards the tibial side is consistent with hip adduction and external rotation.

Digital pivots: They are always consistent with the proximal joint motions and with those of the wrist and hand or the ankle and foot, regardless of the intermediate joint action. In the upper extremity flexion with adduction of fingers occurs with flexion of the wrist and shoulder adduction. Thumb flexion with adduction and internal rotation of the first metacarpal occurs in flexion adduction external rotation pattern. Thumb palmar abduction with abduction and external rotation of the first metacarpal is combined with thumb extension in flexion, abduction, internal rotation pattern. In lower extremity, extension with abduction of the toes is combined with dorsiflexion of the foot and ankle and is consistent with flexion of the hip.

Rotation patterns of neck and upper trunk: They are spiral in character. The major component is one of rotation from extreme left to extreme right or vice versa thereby passing through a flexion phase and into an extension phase. Just as in the diagonal patterns neck rotation is the key to upper trunk rotation.

Line of movement: In the starting position of a given pattern, the major muscle components are in their completely lengthened state, the range of initiation or the stretch range. As a pattern of motion starts, the rotation component enters the motion first as spiral characteristics and other two components combine to give a pattern of diagonal direction. The diagonal line of movement produced by the optimal or maximal contraction of the major muscle components for their lengthened to their shortened stage.

Indications for patterns: Patterns of facilitation are used as passive motion for determination of limitation of range of motion, as free active motion, guided active motion, or resisted motion depending on the indications of exercise. They may be performed through their full range of motion or minimal parts of the motions as indicated. The goal of treatment is the coordinate performance of patterns of facilitation through a full range of motion and with a balance of power between antagonist patterns of both diagonals of motion.

Types of muscle contraction: An attempt by the subject to perform a pattern through a ROM is referred to as active movement with isotonic contraction. When a technique involves an attempt by the subject to hold and part still without permitting ROM to occur it is called as hold or isometric contraction.

1. **Manual contacts:** It uses pressure as a facilitating mechanism. It employs pressure to the groups of muscles tendons and joints responsible for pattern and in the direction to which resistance is to be applied. The physical therapist takes hold of the subject purposefully but without producing painful stimuli. Manual contacts may be varied somewhat with shifting pivots of emphasis and in special situations in order to make pressure more specific in relation to a given muscle or muscle groups. They may be used to place a demand or may be used to give the patient security.
2. **Commands to the subject**: Places a demand on the subject tone of voice may influence considerably the quality of response. Moderate tones should be used when the subject is responding with his best effort and in giving preparatory commands. Strong sharp commands simulate a stress situation and are used when maximal stimulation of active motion is desired as in case of flaccid muscles. Soft tones are

desirable when security is needed by the patients who have symptoms of pain. Action commands must be short accurate and timed to the physical demands. Push, pull are commands for isotonic contraction, hold is the command for isometric contraction and relax or let go are the commands for voluntary relaxation.

3. **Stretch stimulus**: In order to achieve a stretch stimulus in a given pattern, the part must be placed in the extreme lengthened range of that pattern, which is the completely shortened range of the directly antagonistic pattern. The use of the stretch stimulus is helpful in patients having deficiency of innervation. The component of rotation receives first and last consideration, since it is the rotator component which demands complete stretch of all the related muscles in the given pattern. If the maximal stretch is prolonged, adaptation may occur so that the urge to respond with maximal effort is reduced.
4. **Traction and approximation** : They are used to stimulate the proprioceptive centers supplying the joint structures themselves. Either separating the joint structures or compressing the joint surfaces together is helpful means of stimulation. When there is a marked weakness traction or approximation are maintained throughout the active ROM.
5. **Maximal resistance :** It may be defined as greatest amount of resistance which can be applied to an isotonic or active contraction allowing full ROM to occur. When applied to an isometric contraction maximal resistance is the greatest amount which can be applied without defeating or breaking the patients hold. Many mechanical factors involving the relationship of levers axis of motion and the effect of gravity paly a role in determination of amount of resistance given. Resistance may also be graded so as to encourage speed repetition of a motion, conducive to the development of endurance. It is the maximal resistance which provides the means of securing overflow or irradiation from one major muscle component to another.
6. **Normal timing:** It is the sequence of muscle contractions which occurs in any motor activity, resulting in a coordinated movement. Distal to proximal timing is in keeping with the fact that distal parts, the hands and feet, receive most of the stimuli for motor activities. If normal timing in patterns of facilitation has not been developed or deficient it becomes one of the goals of treatment. Proximal deficiencies are corrected first in line with the normal process of development. Distal deficiencies are corrected after proximal control has established.
7. **Timing for emphasis:** It is based upon Beevor's axiom that the brain knows nothing of individual muscles but know only of the movement. In

this maximal resistance is superimposed on patterns of facilitation with due regard for normal timing in order that overflow or irradiation may occur from stronger to weaker muscle components. Timing for emphasis provides the means for increasing response and stimulating action at a specific pivot within a pattern, a specific component in relation to that pivot and a specific part of the range of motion of that pivot.

Techniques of Emphasis

1. **Repeated contractions**: Repetition of activity is necessary to the learning process, the development of strength and endurance. Repeated activity of the weaker major muscle components of a pattern is obtained through a technique of emphasis repeated contractions. By repeating isotonic contractions, the patient may be allowed to work toward the shortened range of pattern. If the initial response was secured in the shortened range, the response may be channeled toward the lengthened range by gradually decreasing the ROM through resistance.
2. **Hold relax active motion:** It provides repetition of isotonic contraction without sustained effort. After eliciting isometric contraction, the patient is asked to relax. As soon as the patient relaxes, the part is taken in the lengthened range and patient is again asked to pull. The procedure is repeated.
3. **Rhythmic stabilization:** It employs isometric contraction of antagonistic and agonistic patterns, which results in cocontraction of antagonists if the isometric contraction is not broken up by the physical therapist. It may be performed at any desired point in the range of motion. Success in application of reversal of antagonists will be dependent on maximal resistance to the antagonists pattern, control of agonists and antagonistic pattern so that the motion can be performed smoothly and careful grading of resistance between the stronger antagonist and weaker agonist. Reversals may be performed in any desired part of the range of motion, which gives the desired response.

Relaxation Techniques

1. **Slow reversal hold relax:** It is a technique of involving an isotonic contraction of the range limiting pattern (the agonistic pattern) followed by an isometric contraction of the antagonistic pattern, followed by a brief period of voluntary relaxation, followed by isotonic contraction

of the agonist pattern. Maximal relaxation is dependent upon maximal resistance applied to the rotation component without allowing range of motion to occur in the other components of the antagonistic pattern.

2. **Contract relax:** In patients presenting marked limitation of range of motion with no active motion available in agonistic pattern, some relaxation of the antagonist pattern may be achieved by using contract relax. This technique involves an isotonic contraction of the antagonist, allowing range of motion in rotation against maxima resistance but no range of the other components, followed by a period of relaxation.
3. **Hold relax:** It is a relaxation technique based on maximal resistance in an isometric contraction. Since no joint motion is implied the technique can be performed as a method of achieving relaxation where muscle spasm is accompanied by pain.
4. **Reinforcement:** Techniques of PNF employ reinforcement as a means of increasing strength of a response. The major muscle components of a specific pattern augment and reinforce each other in order that the motion may be accomplished. The deficient neuromuscular mechanism is incapable of meeting the physical demands of life. This does not preclude the reinforcement of weak patterns by stronger patterns. The less the deficiency, the more effective reinforcement will be. The greater the deficiency, the greater the need for reinforcement. Partial reinforcement may be achieved by having the patient perform a related pattern actively and simultaneously.

BIBLIOGRAPHY

1. Voss DE, Ionta MK. Myess BJ. Proprioceptive neuromuscular facihitation patterns and techniques, 3rd Edn. Philadelphia, Pa: Harper and Row Publishers Inc. 1985.
2. Marek, S, Cramer J, Fincher A, Massey L, Dangelmaier S, Purkayastha S, Acute effects of static and proprioceptive neuromuscular facilitation stretching on muscle strength and power output. J Athlet Train. 2005;40:94-103.
3. McAtee RE, Charland J. Facilitated stretching: assisted and unassisted PNF stretching made easy. 2nd ed. Champaign (IL): Human Kinetics, 1999.
4. Voss DE, Ionta MK, Myers BJ. Proprioceptive neuromuscular facilitation patterns and techniques, 3rd edn. Philadelphia, Pa: Harper and Row Publishers Inc; 1985.
5. Westwater-Wood S, Adams N, Kerry R. The use of proprioceptive neuromuscular facilitation in physiotherapy practice. Physical Therapy Reviews. 2010;15(1):p23-7.

CHAPTER

9

Neural Tissue Mobilization

Learning Objectives

At the end of the chapter learner shall be able to:

1. Describe basic principles.
2. Differentiate between irritable and non-irritable disorder.
3. Enumerate commonly performed techniques.
4. Describe treatment guidelines and treatment progression for irritable disorders.
5. Describe treatment guidelines and treatment progression for non-irritable disorders.

BASIC PRINCIPLES

- The central and peripheral nervous system is a continuous tissue tract that can be considered in three ways (a) Mechanically, the connective tissues are continuous though in different formats, (b) Neurons are interconnected electrically so that the stimulation of the distal most part of the body is perceived by the brain, (c) Chemically, the same neurotransmitters exist centrally and there is flow of cytoplasm inside axons.
- Mechanical features of the nervous system are different from that of other parts of the body. The nervous system is capable of undergoing lengthening during different movements of the body, e.g. it is said that the spinal cord is 5 to 9 cm longer in flexion than in extension.
- Gross shape and features of central and peripheral nervous system are so framed that it can perform two important functions such as

uninterrupted impulse conduction and support and protection of impulse conducting tissue.

- The mechanical interface: It may be defined as that tissue or material adjacent to the nervous system that can move independently of the system (Butler 1989). Although a pure mechanical interface may be a fascial sheet or a blood vessel, a more relevant interface such as muscle or ligament adjacent to it.
- Nervous system adaptations to movement take place by lengthening and shortening during the movement. There occurs increased intradural or intraneural pressure. Intraneural movement occurs due to movement of the neural tissue elements in relation to the connective tissue interfaces. But there are certain points where no nervous system movement occurs in relation to the interface. These are called as Tension Points. According to Louis (1981) the C6, T6 and L4 vertebral levels some of the examples of tension points. These are also the points where the extraneural vessels enter the nervous system in areas of little movement relative to the interface. Thus in general there is a link between anatomy, biomechanics and blood supply of nervous system.
- Whenever there is injury to the nervous system, vascular and mechanical factors play an important role in clinical picture.
  - Vascular factors: Nerve fibers are dependent on uninterrupted blood supply for normal functioning. With injury to the nervous system there occurs venous stasis and consequent hypoxia. This results in impaired nerve fiber nutrition. Neuroischemia is likely to be a source of pain and other symptoms such as paresthesia.
  - Mechanical factors: Mechanical changes in the interface in a segment of a nervous system will alter tension in whole of the nervous system. This alteration in tension results in appearance of symptoms in other areas where initially there was no injury.

The ultimate aim of the treatment is to restore the patient's range of nervous system movement and stretch capabilities and to normalize the sensitivity of the system. This technique is more difficult than joint mobilization and manipulation. There are no bony levers to push on and it is more difficult to visualize than non-neural structures. Management of all disorders involves some consideration of the nervous system. Even if the injury is non-neural, the nervous system is the pathway for expression of the symptoms and motor output such as muscle spasm and autonomic reactions.

There are situations where the nervous system is clearly involved and is the dominant structure in a disorder. Archnoiditis or acute nerve root compression are examples. There are others where the mechanical shortcomings of the system are just part of the disorder, for example, dural sleeve irritation in the presence of a gross foraminal stenosis.

Disorders suitable for mobilization can be very broadly separated into those whose origin may result from a biomechanical compromise (pathomechanics) or an inflammatory reaction (pathophysiology). The entrapped nerve or abnormally tethered dural ligaments are examples of the former. Intraneural swellings and irritated dura are examples of the latter. These two situations will invariably, although one will predominate and consequently determine the emphasis in management. A pathophysiological situation could lead to a pathomechanical squeal.

TENSION TESTING

Examination and treatment with NTM often involve derivation from the base tests. These base tests are:

- Passive neck flexion (PNF)
- Straight leg raise(SLR)
- Slump test
- Prone knee bend (PKB)
- Upper limb tension tests (ULTT)

Passive Knee Flexion (PNF)

With patient in supine lying position , patient is asked to flex his neck as much as possible. After active movement, the therapist passively flexes the neck till chin on chest position. The symptom responses, range of movement and resistance felt during the test are noted. Normally, the movement is painless except a stretching pain. PNF is indicated in all possible spinal disorders. It may also be indicated for headache symptoms and for arm and leg pain of spinal origin. Senstisiation can be done by: a) Side-lying position; b) Thoracic flexion.

Passive knee extension is done when there is a high level of suspicion of adverse tension in a disorder or the subjective complaints of the patient indicate that the cervical extension is an involved movement in the disorder. PNF alters not only cervical and thoracic spine, but also alters lumbar spine mechanics. If PNF produces lumbar pain, it can be inferred that the source of that pain lies within the nervous system or in a pathological relationship with the structures to which it is attached.

Straight Leg Raise (SLR)

With the patient in supine lying, trunk and hips in neutral position , examiner places one hand at the heel and the other hand behind the knee joint. Examiner asks for any base line symptoms if present. Examiner lifts the leg up with the knee in extension up to a point where patient complains of increased symptoms or available ROM. It is important for an examiner to note symptom response and resistance encountered through the movement. These responses on the affected side are compared with that on the normal side. Pillow should not be used testing, but if it is used the same pillow should be given during the reassessment. This is important because the position of cervical region has an important effect on SLR.

Normally, the range of motion available without any adverse symptoms is 70–80°

It is not only the degree of movement that is only important but it should be interpreted along with the symtoms response, the SLR range of the contralateral limb and the overall patient presentation. Other postural

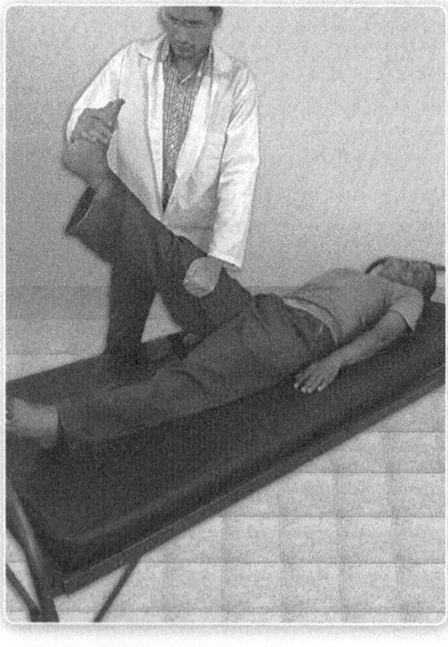

Fig. 9.1: Straight leg raise

responses such as neck flexion, extension or side flexion, extension of the contralater limb should also be noted.

It should be routinely done for all patients with spinal and leg pain. there are various sensitizing maneuvers that needs to be added depending on the patients response. The most commonly used sensitizing additions are ankle dorsiflexion (DF), ankle plantar flexion inversion/(PF/I), hip adduction, hip medial rotation and passive neck flexion (PNF). This addition can be done before the base test is completed or after the base test is completed. The best response will be gained if movements at the site of tension are taken up first. It can be noted by adding.

Dorsiflexion of ankle joint can be added to basic SLR for sensitizing the nervous tissue further. If symptoms are more in the region of Achillis tendon then dorsiflexion can be added first. Dorsiflexion added to SLR would be a useful sensitizer if could alter the spinal symptoms provoked by SLR. It can be further sensitized by adding eversion of the foot, extension of toes and stretching the plantar fascia, it places more tension on tibial tract. If inversion is added, it places tension along the sural nerve.

Ankle plantarflexion and inversion will add tension along the common peronela tract. It can also be added before after the basic SLR test. This addition is of great clinical value in the examination of disorders such as shin splints or chronic ankle sprain.

Hip adduction: Sciatic nerve being lateral to ischial tuberosity addition of adduction will add further tension to the nervous system. The same range SLR must be maintained when hip adduction is being added.

Hip medial rotation: It will further sensitize the sciatic nerve. So addition of hip medial rotation to SLR will worsen the spinal/leg symptoms. It probably sensitise the common peroneal division more than the tibial division of the sciatic nerve.

Addition of cervical flexion to a SLR would change the symptom response and range of movement of SLR. The SLR response would be different if CF is added before or after the test. So the same maneuver should be repeated during reassessment. Cervical extension can also be added as a sensitizing maneuver.

Bowstring test: The hip is flexed to the point of response and then lowered to the point just short of response. If at his point pressure on tibial nerve in the popliteal fossa makes the symptoms worse than the test is positive. Crossed SLR when the unaffected leg is lifted up is said to be positive when there is reproduction of the symptoms. It is the best indicator of the disc prolapse.

Prone Knee Bend (PKB)

With the patient in prone position, head rotated toward the therapist who is standing on one side of the patient the examiner grasps the lower leg and flexes the knee to a predetermined symptom response. Note should be taken regarding the type of symptom response and resistance felt throughout ROM. Normally, patient is able to touch the heel to the buttock with some difficulty. Compensatory.strategies such as lifting up of the buttock is also seen to consider the test to positive patient should complain of pain on anterior aspect of thigh, knee joint or upper lumbar region.

Further sensitization can be done by extending the hip joint. Positive test may indicate Meralgia Paresthetica. Hip adduction may be further added to PKB/HE. Slump test may be added to PKB in side-lying position. This is done to allow differentiation of nervous system involvement from non-nervous system structures (Fig. 9.2).

Slump Test

With the patient in high sitting position, thighs fully supported, hands of patient are behind the back. Resting symptoms should be noted. Following steps are done: Ask the patient to sag his back with the neck in neutral position, apply overpressure at the thoracic and lumbar spine, ask the patient to bend his neck with chin-to-chest position, active extension

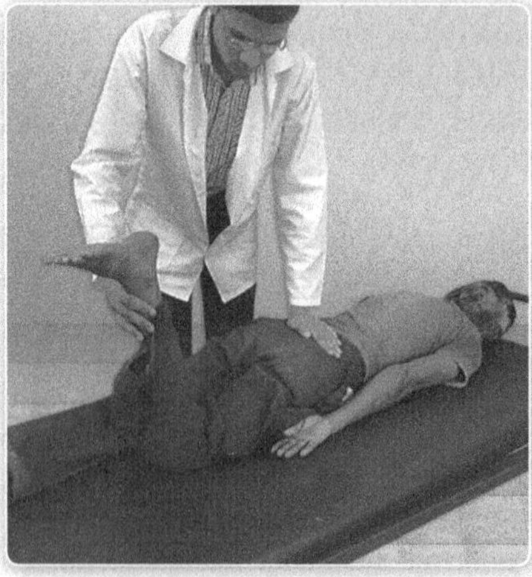

Fig. 9.2: Prone knee bending

of the knee (sound side first), dorsiflexion of ankle (sound side first), release neck flexion. Same procedure is repeated with the other leg. The range of movement and pain responses are compared.

The most important precaution while performing the test is that the whole test may not be performed totally at one sitting. Symptom response will govern whether the next step should be added or not, i.e. if patient complains of increased symptoms at any stage , then the next step should not be performed.

Normally patient may complain of stretch pain on extension of knee and ankle dorsiflexion and decrease in these symptoms on release of neck. But a patient with discogenic disorder will complain of increased symptoms at any stage. The obturator nerve can be tested by abducting the leg in slump position.

Slump test can also be performed in long sitting position. With the patient in long sitting position, feet against the wall to add dorsiflexion, trunk flexion is done, followed by neck flexion. Symptom response to every stage is noted. This test is specially indicated in those patients who complain of symptoms in long sitting position (Fig. 9.3).

Upper Limb Tension Test-1 (ULTT-1)

With the patient in supine lying, examiner places one hand on the top of the shoulder. A constant depression force is applied with this hand.

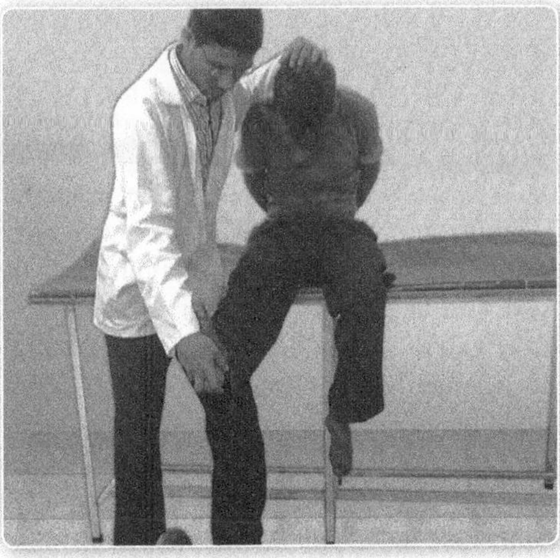

Fig. 9.3: Slump test

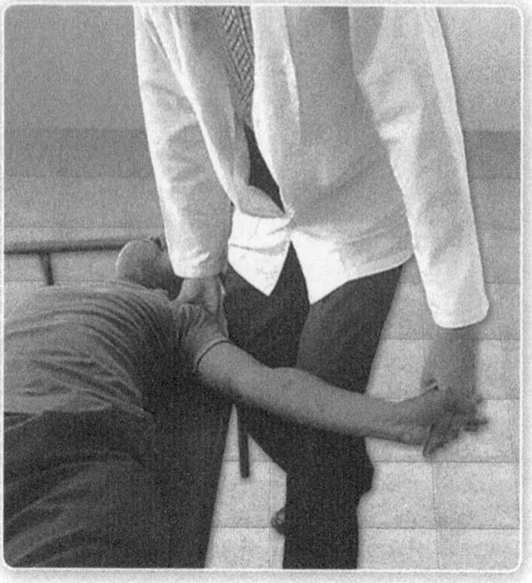

Fig. 9.4: Upper limb tension test-1

With the other hand on the ventral aspect of the patient's hand, examiner performs abduction of shoulder to 110°. Then the forearm is supinated and wrist and fingers are extended. The shoulder is laterally rotated and elbow is extended. With this position of UE, cervical lateral flexion to left and right should be added. Proper instructions should be given to the patient for lateral flexion of the neck. As with other testing, symptom response and resistance should be noted during the testing.

It is indicated for all patients with symptoms anywhere in the arm, head, neck and thoracic spine. Normally, the patient would complain of a deep stretch or ache in the cubital fossa.

UPPER LIMB TENSION TEST-2 (ULTT-2)

For left UE, with the patient lying supine, the examiner's right hand holds patient's elbow and left hand holds patients's wrist. Due to this crossed arm position therapist will require minimal changes during the maneuver and the technique will be better controlled. With the thigh resting against the patient's shoulder, examiner carefully depresses the patient's shoulder girdle. It is followed by extension of the patient's elbow, lateral rotation of shoulder, pronation of forearm, extension of wrist, fingers and thumb. For radial nerve bias shoulder is medially rotated, wrist is flexed. Further flexion of the thumb and ulnar deviation will further sensitize the radial nerve.

UPPER LIMB TENSION TEST-3

Position of patient and examiner is same as that for ULTT1. With the patient in supine position, patient's wrist is extended and forearm supinated. It is followed by flexion of the elbow , shoulder depression, shoulder abduction. It is an ulnar nerve bias test.

Precautions

- There may occur damage to other structures involved in testing since tension tests are complex they involve many components that are often spread all over the body. So other structures could be injured or aggravated by the testing itself, e.g. during ULTT when neck movements are introduced, the injured zygapophyseal joints may further be damaged.
- Irritability: It indicates acuteness of the disorder. If the condition is irritable, utmost precaution should be taken while adding various components to the basic tests.
- Behavior of symptoms: If the disorder is worsening rapidly, then due precaution should be taken while assessing with tension tests. Physical handling of the patient whose symptoms has progressed rapidly needs to be careful enough.
- Unstable neurological signs: If the disorder is acute then the utmost precaution needs to be taken while performing tension tests.
- General health problems: Great respect should be given to pathologies affect the nervous system, although manual treatment may be appropriate for some of the symptoms evoked.
- Dizziness: Nervous system mobilization may be a risk factor for mobilizing the cervical spine with minimal interference to joints and vertebral joints. Also dizziness related to vertebrobasillary insufficiency is a contraindication to cervical manipulation .
- Circulatory disturbances: It is well known that while mobilizing nervous system, the circulatory system which is closely connected with nervous sytem also gets mobilized. Hence due care should be taken if there are any signs of circulatory disturbances.
- Frank cord injury: Extra care should be taken if the patient is diagnosed with cord damage. With mobilization or testing it may be possible that cord may get injured further.

Contraindications

- Recent onset of, or worsening of neurological signs: Acute conditions which are unstable enough to require daily neurological examination are an absolute contraindication to mobilization to nervous system.
- Cauda equina lesions: Bladder and bowel problem or dysfunction due to cauda equine lesion could be a surgical emergency and hence is a contraindication for mobilization of the nervous system.
- Injury to the spinal cord: When a cord is tethered to the dura mater which may in turn be tethered to the spinal canal, is an absolute contraindication for a nervous system mobilization.

Treatment Guidelines

It is convenient to discuss disorders in the categories of irritable- (pathophysiological) and nonirritable disorders (pathomechanical dominance).

The treatment of the signs, symptoms based on severity irritability and nature of the disorder in accordance with the Maitland concept. Similar grading system is used for giving the treatment.

- Grade I—small amplitude movement at the beginning of the range of motion (ROM).
- Grade II—Large amplitude movement in the mid range of movement.
- Grade III—Small amplitude movement at the end of the available ROM
- Grade IV—Small amplitude movement near the end ROM stressing into the tissue resistance.

Irritable disorder: This is the example of a disorder where the initial considerations in the treatment of the nervous system component must be directed towards pathophysiology. Assessing the contributions of each structure to symptoms and the relative importance of treatment to each structure can be difficult. In an irritable disorder, there are advantages in being able to move one structure without interfering too much with others in the local area.

Guidelines for starting technique: A technique well removed from the symptom area is applicable. Thus neural structures can therefore be mobilized in the injured area and the non-neural structures only minimally moved. The technique should be non-provoking initially, thus remaining short of any increase in symptoms. It is best to under treat initially until the sensitivity of the neural component of the disorder becomes apparent. Suggested grades of techniques are large amplitude grade IIs performed slowly and rhythmically through range with maximal respect to symptoms. Grade IV techniques just nudging at resistance with similar respect for symptoms are also a possibility. In performing grade II, it is recommended that largest amplitude possible should be done.

It is necessary in case of irritable disorders that the symptoms are continuously monitored. For this, a constant verbal and nonverbal communication must be made with the patient. A constant ache or increase in the constant ache should be avoided. If at all, it is acceptable for some symptoms that the symptoms can be allowed to reappear, they should be rhythmic with the technique, i.e. on and off rather than continuous.

Patient should be positioned optimally comfortable and relaxed so that the optimum recovery of the nervous system in relation interfacing tissues. This can be accomplished by positioning the patient in pain relieving position. Muscle is the most common interfacing tissue, which may have an effect on the status of pain. If these are contracted, it is possible that the sliding of neural structures is impaired. Passive movement of the nervous system can be given in a very gentle manner if the disorder is deemed to be less irritable. Or technique may move closer to the source of symptoms. Rest is also important in the treatment though it can be biased in a way the anti-tension positioning may be adopted by the patient, which may possible lead to relief of symptoms.

Treatment progression: There is an infinite number of ways and directions in which techniques can be applied to influence the nervous system.

The number of repetitions can be increased. In the irritable disorder we prefer to perform a sequence of gentle oscillations may be 20 per second and reassess the effect. The amplitude can also be increased. The technique could be progressed to a point where some symptoms are reproduced or it could be taken to a point where some resistance to the movement is encountered.

The technique could be repeated with the nervous system in more tension. Knee extension hip flexion could be performed initially with spine in neutral position and progressed to with spine in some amount of flexion.

The application of the technique can be moved closer to the symptom area.

The continuum of the nervous system also allows easy regression of a technique. So, if the symptoms are being provoked by one technique, it can be replaced by another technique in the same region or that same technique needs to be performed more gently. Another alternative can be that the technique be performed in less tension.

Treatment of the Non-irritable Disorders

Duration of the disorder has an effect on the use of structures and problems arise due to disuse and the products of an inflammatory response giving a picture of a pathomechanical nature. Hence to tackle such a problem of pathomechanical nature, one needs to utilize the techniques that address the mechanics. Mechanically-based treatment is the best way to treat a mechanical problem of the nervous system.

Guidelines for Starting the Technique

The treatment may be directed at other tissues such as stiff lumbar joints to relieve the tension on neural structures. To begin with the initial technique should be in the grade III and/or grade IV. Stressing into the tissue resistance is necessary as it alters the mechanics. If irritability is a concern then the initially the technique may be non-provoking but later on it would include some amount of discomfort. In grade III mobilization, there occurs considerable nervous system movement in relation to the interfacing structures with a short low dose tension at the end of range for a given period. Conversely, grade IV maintains tension at the end of range with little or no movement of the nervous system.

When there are abnormalities of mechanics of the nervous system in relation with the interface (extraneural), grade III mobilization techniques which are through range, large amplitude movement are preferred. In case of injury reactions which are intraneural in nature, small amplitude movements with the nervous system on some stretch are used. But as a rule, any symptoms that are provoked during the treatment should subside immediately when the treatment technique is released. Irritability will play an important role in choosing the technique. In case if the condition is irritable, It may be desirable to keep a component away from the source of symptoms initially.

Treatment Progression

Following are the ways in which the treatment can be progressed:

- Duration of a hold can be increased. The starting technique can be performed for a longer period. Alternatively it can be stressed more into the resistance which may result in provocation of the symptoms.

- Basic starting position can be repeated with other components in some other different positions. This will usually involve an increase in overall nervous system tension.
- The movement can be done more closely to the symptom area.
- As a progression of treatment of non-neural structures involved in this disorder, these structures can be treated in a tension position, e.g. in slump position, unilateral posteroanterior pressure over a rib or a zygoapophyseal joint can be given.

Following points needs to be taken into consideration while treating non-irritable disorders.

- Selection of the technique: If the base tests are used as the treatment, then more vigor will usually be required to correctly access the nervous system than if the technique involved movements which produce signs and symptoms more easily. For example if ULTT1 is used as a treatment technique for mechanical symptoms in cervical region, to be effective enough at the cervical spine with less force, the cervical spine should be in some amount of lateral flexion along with some sensitizing maneuver of ULTT1 such as wrist extension or elbow extension should be added. Also, the greater the concern about irritability of the disorder, oscillatory techniques are used.
- Number of repetitions: To determine this, clinical reasoning skills are required. One needs to answer how many, how much, how long. Any technique should not be sustained for more than 10 seconds. In the less irritable disorder where pathomechanics is a concern, one or two firm repetitions of a technique needs to be performed.
- Continuum of the nervous system: In most adverse tension disorders, there will be axial and transverse tension considerations. It should be clear that if a person is to have optimum upper limb tension tests they will require an optimum slump and vice versa. They will also require an optimum ULTT of the other arm.
- Immediate effect: With nervous system mobilization in non-irritable disorder, no matter how strong is the treatment, the symptoms reproduced disappear within seconds of stopping. This is most likely to be due to replenishment of blood to the nerve fibers rendered hypoxic by stretch or compression.
- Reassessment: It is important to know the behavior of symptoms during and after the treatment session. It is not uncommon that a patient to report of increased pain in some other region after the treatment is over. This is because if a tension is altered in one area, an altered tension and nervous system relationship with interfacing structures may be set

up elsewhere. This may be symptom provocative and take some time for the patient to adjust to. If on reassessment, it is found that there is no improvement, and then the technique should not be continued.

BIBLIOGRAPHY

1. Butler DS, Mobilisation of the nervous system. Melbourne, Churchill Livingstone, 1991.
2. Gifford L. Neurodynamics. In: Pitt-Brooke J, Reid H, Lockwood J, Kerr K, (Eds). Rehabilitation of movement. London, UK: WB Saunders Company Ltd; 1998. pp. 159-95.
3. Maitland GD vertebral manipulation, 5th edition, Butterworths, London.
4. Shacklock MO. Clinical applications of neurodynamics. In: Shacklock MO, (Ed) editor. Moving in on Pain. Chatswood, UK: Butterworth-Heinemann; 1995. pp. 123-131.
5. Shacklock MO. Neurodynamics. Physiotherapy. 1995;81:9-16.

CHAPTER

10

Cyriax's Deep Friction Massage

Learning Objectives

At the end of the chapter learner shall be able to:

1. Define deep transverse friction.
2. Describe the mode of action.
3. Enlist indications and contraindications.
4. Explain clinical reasoning behind each indication and contraindication.
5. Enumerate the steps in treatment.
6. Describe the technique in detail.

DEEP TRANSVERSES FRICTION

It was derived by Cyriax. It implies massage applied by fingers directly to the lesion and transverse to the direction of fibers. It can be used after a injury or for mechanical overuse in muscular tendinous and ligamentous structures. Friction is usually slower in effect than injection but produce more fundamental resolution of the lesion resulting in permanent cure and less recurrence. It is vital that deep friction be performed at the exact site of lesion. The effect is so local that unless the finger is applied at the exact site and friction given in right direction, relief cannot be expected. In minor muscular tears friction is usually followed by active movements, in ligamentous tears by passive movement and in tendinous lesions by avoidance of the painful activity until full resolution has been achieved.

MODE OF ACTION

Friction has a local anti-inflammatory and pain diminishing effect and results in a better alignment of connective tissue fibrils.

Reduction of post-traumatic inflammation: Deep massage diminishes excessive post-traumatic inflammation and facilitates free use of the injured part. This is partly as an outcome of local traumatic hyperemia as a result of mechanical increase in blood supply.

Relief of pain: Deep massage has a pain relieving effect due to neurogenic influences and/or according to Cyriax to increased destruction of Lewes' substance p. This metabolite if present in large quantity may lead to ischemia and pain stimulation of the mechanoreceptors of the affected structures by deep friction consequently leads to reduced pain sensation. Friction results in an immediate pain diminishing effect and progressive further decrease in pain during the weeks of treatment. The temporary relief at the end of the session permits other treatment not otherwise possible such as manipulation rupture of adhesions.

Prevention and breaking of adhesions: Friction has an effect on connective tissue in that it prevents or ruptures abnormal crosslinks and adhesions. Whereas long friction only increases the blood flow and lymph, transverse friction moves the tissue fibers on each other and in relation to adjacent structures in imitation of their natural behavior. Because stretching is avoided, no stress falls on the (tissues) site of healing or the scar tissue being formed. In ligamentous, tendons and muscle belies the fibers have a long course and lesions usually results from axial overstretching.

From the second day of injury new collagen fibers begin to fill the gap. Initially these fibers are disorderly in that the affected structure is usually held immobile because of pain. At this stage cross linkage between fibers is present but the matrix is still very fragile and weak and can be a easily disrupted. When friction stresses begin, the collagen fibers that are produced orient along the line of force. In consequence, movement ensures orderly deposition of new fibrils and prevents inappropriate cross linkages. Therefore, during the healing period, the affected structures should be kept mobile by using them normally.

However, because of a severe inflammatory reaction as in acute ligamentous lesions the joint cannot be moved to the full extent actively and so movement between bone and ligament is restricted. This problem can be solved by friction. When given transverse to the direction, normal mobility between the affected fibers and neighboring structures such as normal tissue fibers and bone prevents bone formation.

Transverse friction also assists fibroblast orientation. In the early stages of fibroblast proliferation when cross links are weak or absent, friction must be very light so as to cause minimal discomfort. Therefore during the initial period of 24–48 hours, friction is given with a very light pressure and over a short duration say one minute. Later if strong cross links or adhesion have been more intense friction is needed to break these down. Sometimes when adhesion with neighboring structures have already been formed, manipulative rupture may be required.

Indication

Diagnosis: Friction may help to define the exact site. A few minutes of massage on the lesion results in diminished pain on testing immediately thereafter, so confirming the diagnosis as accurately or more accurately.
Preparation for using other technique: For reasons of pain relief, transverse massage is usually required before manipulative rupturing of ligament adhesions is performed. This may be indicated at the MCL at the knee or LCL of the ankle.
Therapy:

i. *Muscle bellies:* Friction is given to a muscle belly in contusion, in lesions due to repeated overuse in myosynovitis and after a minor muscular tear which may be the result of one major strain or of repeated overuse. Transverse friction mobilizes the longitudinal muscle fibers without pulling on the tear so preventing (in the early stage) or breaking down (in the chronic stage) abnormal crosslinks.

   To break down cross links, friction is given forcefully and for a duration of 15–20 minutes. Prophylactic friction is more gently applied for shorter duration.

   Friction to a muscle belly is always given with the muscle well relaxed. In a recent minor tear, friction is followed by active contraction with the muscle in position of maximal relaxation and without weight bearing so that no tension falls on the healing breach. To avoid recurrence, friction is given for 1 week beyond the time at which all clinical tests have become negative. During whole of treatment period all movements or activities that bring on pain should be avoided by the patient.

ii. *Musculotendinous junction:* Those musculotendinous junctions which have both muscular and tendinous fibers throughout the whole body can be treated by deep transverse friction.

iii. *Tendons:* All mechanical tendinitis and tenosynovitis can be treated by deep massage except for tenoperiosteal origin of ECRB.

In tenosynovitis occurring in long tendons with a sheath, roughening of the gliding surfaces of both tendon and sheath give rise to pain and sometimes to crepitus. Because limitation of movement is not found, adhesions do not occur. The condition is the result of longitudinal friction between the tendon and sheath so friction perpendicular to the line of mechanical effect, i.e. transverse, has a curative action useful in both chronic and acute conditions. Manual rolling of the tendon sheath over and against the tendon smoothes off the roughened surfaces. For maximal efficacy the tendon with its sheath must be put under tension during massage so that the tendon forms an immobile base against which the tendon sheath is moved. In tendinitis of tendons without a sheath a painful scar in the tendon body or at the tenoperiosteal insertion may follow respective overuse or a sudden strain.

These lesions if not too extensive can be treated by steroid infiltration but the recurrence is about one in five. Therefore, it may be better to treat them by deep friction which require more time but breaks up the abnormal scar tissue and therefore it leads to more definite healing and with less chances of recurrence.

During the whole period of treatment of tendinitis, tenosynovitis, the patient must avoid all activities that provoke the pain.

iv. *Ligaments:* Most ligaments allow movement between the bones they link and after a sprain this mobility must be conserved. Newly formed fibers of scar tissue lying longitudinally, i.e. in the same direction as the original fibers are beneficial whereas adhesions to the underlying structures disturb normal function and must be prevented or broken down.

In recent ligament sprains, local swelling is removed as much as possible by effleurage which is proximally directed over skin and underlying soft tissues. It is followed by friction of short duration say 1 minute and low intensity for the first two days, with the ligament somewhat under tension. As the pain diminishes over subsequent days the intensity of friction is progressively increased to about 4–5 minutes for 2–3 days and finally to a full duration of 15–20 minutes from the third day. Friction is followed by passive and active movements within the limits of pain to maintain normal gliding of the ligament over adjacent bones.

v. *Joint capsules:* Arthritis of the trapezium 1st CMC joint, TMJ and cervical facet joints can be treated by deep friction if arthritis is not too advanced.

Contraindications

i. Ossification and calcification of soft tissues and extensive ossification in muscle, tendons ligaments or capsules is a bar to all active treatment. In supraspinatus tendinitis, calcification is regarded as responsible for complaints. When insertion is tender to touch and radiographs shows calcification. These findings are contraindication to friction. In contrast when calcification is present in the absence of severe tenderness transverse massage can be given.
ii. Bacterial Rheumatoid type tendinitis.
iii. Skin problem such as ulcers psoriasis and blisters.
vi. Neighboring bacterial infection.
v. Bursitis and disorders of nerve structures.

Technique

Massage can only reach deep seated structures if deep friction technique of Cyriax is used. In that, it implies a very precise technique. Attention must be paid to different elements such as the position of patient and of the therapist hand, which fingers are used, the amount of pressure, the duration and frequency of the sessions. It is essential that the therapeutic movement is confined to the lesion which may occupy only a small volume.

In some instances, it will be necessary to palpate carefully the entire structure at fault so as to find the most tender spot which indicate the lesion. The patient's skin and therapist's finger must move as one so that the deep layers of the skin move over the affected bone.

The massage is unpleasant as the digits rub across muscle tendon or ligament but it should not be painful. About 6 to 12 treatment sessions are normally needed.

Except in ligament disorders they are not given more often than every other day because otherwise the site of lesion may still be too tender from the previous treatment to permit adequate massage.

Position of the Patient

The patient's position must be comfortable because it need to maintain for 15–20 minutes. Sitting or lying are preferable.

The lesion must be brought within finger's reach. In addition, the affected structures must be under some optimum of tension. While positioning the patient full relaxation is necessary for a muscle belly in order not only to treat its surface but also to access the deeply seated lesion. Tendons with a sheath must be kept taut otherwise friction will be ineffective between tendon and sheath.

The same applies in ligamentous lesion which are also placed in tension within the limits of pain.

Position of the Therapist and his Hands

The bodily position of the therapist must be most comfortable and least tiring in that while the patient is present for perhaps half an hour, the therapist is in action for a whole day. Working heights is of chief importance so an adjustable high low couch is ideal.

The majority of friction techniques are performed in two phases an active movement usually as a result of the muscular activity and a passive movement when the arm and hand is returned to a starting position. In the end of passive movement, there should also be a moment of rest during which the therapist fully relaxes the muscle. The larger and stronger muscle should always be used. Flexor activity usually includes muscle of both arm and hand. The therapist should use one set of muscle to apply the pressure on a specific area and another set of muscle to provide movement. For example,. pressure can be given with fingers and movement can be given with arm.

The shoulder should not be abduction because this quickly leads to pain and cramp in the deltoid. Digits, hand and forearm muscle should generally form a straight line and are kept parallel to the direction of movement. The position of hands depends on the tissue to be treated and the surface worked on. In principle, they should rest on the patient's body and movement performed should be as natural as possible. The wrist and MTP joints should be kept in an almost neutral position. The interphalangeal joints are slightly flexed. The finger position depends on whether the fingers are used to provide counter pressure or to perform the massage.

Counter Pressure

Counter pressure is usually provided to enable a good sweep. The fingers applying counter pressure and stabilization are most impatient in bringing those applying friction into the right position also determining the direction of friction. The thumb is used when massage is performed with the index finger reinforced by the middle fingers or middle aided by index finger when the thumb does the massage and the counter pressure is from the fingers. Sometimes the counter pressure is not given- when supine promotion movements are given to the anterior aspect of Achiles tendon, in to and fro movements as in friction to the quadriceps expansion and on rolling movements as in friction to the populates muscle belly. The most common way of applying friction around a round edge on a flat surface is to use index reinforced by the middle finger. Sometimes the opposite is done, i.e. the middle finger is reinforced by index. This technique is often used where the lesion is different to reach, i.e quadriceps expansion at the knee. It is also useful for the pronation/ supination because middle finger is longest, e.g. in upper part of tibialis posterior, ant aspect of Achilles tendon and the interosseous muscle of the hand.

In rather large lesion as in peroneal tendinitis two or three adjacent fingers are used together. The thumb perform friction in deep seated lesions as in long head of biceps in bicipital groove. For muscle belly lesion, the affected part is taken between thumb and finger in a pinching grip. Sometimes the same technique is used in tendinous lesions, e.g. at the sides of the Achiles tendon.

No Movement between Finger and Skin is Allowed

Deep friction can only be effective when skin and subcutaneous fascia are moved over tendon ligaments or muscle. No movement is allowed between the therapists' finger and patients skin blistering soon take place and usually indicates faulty techniques.

Sometimes, it can be avoided by keeping the skin dry by the use of 95% alcohol in water and or by placing a piece of cotton in between the finger and the skin.

In the obese subcutaneous soreness and/or ecchymosis occasionally occurs and sometimes a nodule may form. For this reason, the finger should not be in continuous contact with the same area but displace the skin to one or the other side before applying pressure.

Direction of Friction must be Transverse to the tissue Fibers

Longitudinal massage improves the circulation of blood and lymph but has no effect on muscular skeletal lesion. To restore or to maintain mobility of a lesion massage must be given across the fibers so moving all fibers in relation to each other. To achieve this, the therapist must have a good anatomical knowledge of the direction of fibers.

Sweep

The main goal of friction is to move the fibers in relation to each other and adjacent structures enough sweep must be given to the friction for this purpose so the friction starts at the far side of the lesion, glides over it and ends at the near edge. Adequate sweep is sometimes limited by the amount and elasticity of the over lying skin. Initial displacement of skin over the lesion from near to the far side may help increase the sweep and reduce the risk of blistering.

Amount of Pressure: It Depends on

1. The depth of lesion: The friction must always reach the sufficient depth to move the affected fibers in relation to their neighbors and sometimes the underlying bone or capsule. Increased pressure must be applied to the deeper structures.
2. Age of lesion: Recent sprains require only preventive friction because crosslinks or adhesions have not had time to form. In long standing cases, more pressure is needed to get rid of these. However, pressure should always be associated with movement and should not replace it because pressure alone is in effective and but it is painful.
3. The tenderness of the tension: In severely inflamed lesions that are very tender to touch, friction with the usual amount of force may be painful. Pain can be avoided by starting with minimum amount of pressure just enough to reach the lesion and progressively increasing the force as the treatment proceeds.

Duration and Frequency

Friction is usually given for 10–20 minutes and because of tenderness on every second day, the ideal timing the next treatment is when local tenderness caused by the previous session has resolved. If tenderness persists after 2 days, the pressure used during friction should not be diminished but the interval between the sessions must be increased. Massage immediately after a ligament sprain or a minor muscular rupture may be applied daily for the first weak, but should be of very low intensity and short duration.

Treatment is stopped once the patient is pain free during daily activities and functional tests are totally negative. Local tenderness may persist longer but disappears spontaneously because it is the outcome of repetitive hard pressure. However, in a minor lesion of a muscle belly massage is continued for 1 week after full clinical recovery to prevent recurrence.

BIBLIOGRAPHY

1. Bulckwater JA, Crues R. Healing of musculoskeletal tissues. In : Rockwood CA, Green DP (Eds). Fractures, JP Lipincott, Philadelphia 1991.
2. Chamberlain G. Cyriax's friction massage: A review. J Orthop Sports Phys Ther. 1982. 4:16-22
3. Woodman RM, Pare L. Evaluation and treatment of soft tissue lesions of the ankle and forefoot using the Cyriax approach. Physical Therapy. 1982. 62:1144-7

CHAPTER

11

McKenzie's Approach

Learning Objectives

At the end of this chapter the learner shall be able to:

1. Define Syndrome.
2. Enumerate the three types of syndrome.
3. Describe the clinical features of these syndromes.
4. Describe the traffic light principle.
5. Describe management for each syndrome.

According to McKenzie, syndrome is defined as a set of signs and symptoms that collectively characterize a particular disease or abnormal condition. It implies that the actual cause is unknown.

There are three main types of pain syndrome:

Mechanical spinal pain is caused by mechanical deformation of soft tissues containing nociceptive receptors. McKenzie states that all spinal mechanical pain can be classified into three syndromes: the postural, dysfunction and derangement syndrome.

a. **Postural syndrome:** Postural pain appears after prolonged static loading, which in turn causes overstretching and mechanical deformation of normal spinal tissue. The pain eases and then stops on removal of the loading.
b. **Dysfunction syndrome:** Dysfunctional pain appears immediately when shortened spinal tissues are mechanically deformed by overstretching. The pain eases and then stops on removal of end range stress.

c. **Derangement syndrome:** Derangement pain is felt immediately or eventually when there is an anatomical disruption or displacement of the intervertebral segment.

Predisposing factors of mechanical spinal pain: McKenzie states that there are two most significant factors which are prolonged poor sitting posture and frequency of flexion in people's lifestyle.

Prolonged sitting: Sitting with lumbar kyphosis increases low back and referred pain as compared to sitting with lordiosis. The lordotic posture also shows a significant shift of the most peripheral pain towards the low back.

Frequency of flexion: It is directly proportional to the gradual disc prolapse and annular failure following prolonged flexion loading as described by Adams (1985) on cadaveric specimens. Eventually supportive soft tissues succumb to these stresses of poor sitting and sustained flexion and fail without being subject to violent external forces.

THE POSTURAL SYNDROME

Definition: In postural syndrome patients complains of pain because they are mechanically deforming their spinal soft tissue due to sustaining end range postures and positions.

Pain in this syndrome is caused due to prolonged static loading of soft tissues contained within or adjacent to the spinal column. In the cervical spine this mainly occurs due to poor sitting posture where in the neck is continuously placed in protruded position. This causes shortening of the posterior structures in the neck region. Also in lying position, end range rotation and side flexion occurs. In the lumbar spine postural pain occurs when the lumbar spine is kept at end range flexion in prolonged sitting or bending forwards or when the low lumbar spine is in sustained extension as occurs with relaxed standing.

Patients suffering from postural syndrome are usually under 30 years of age, sedentary workers who are not doing regular exercises in any form. It has an insidious onset and gradually worsens over a period of time.

Pain is felt locally and symmetrically usually adjacent to the midline of the spine in the cervicothoracic junction and in the mid thoracic and low lumbar region. It is often accompanied by a headache. The pain is not continuous and patient complains of pain only when a stretch is placed on the tightened structures which are under prolonged stress. This may also be associated with increased pain as the day progresses. Also pain may alter with change in position, with certain positions it may disappear totally.

Aim of treatment in such patients is to correct the posture which will result in relieving of the passive tension placed on the tissues.

Dysfunction Syndrome

In this, patients complain of pain when there is a mechanical deformation of the previously shortened structures within or surrounding the spine. Pain may also be felt when patient attempts end range movement. Dysfunction may also mean loss of joint play (Mennell) which can be due to adaptive shortening, contracture, scarring, adherence or fibrosis.

In dysfunction, the soft tissues within or surrounding the involved spinal segment are shortened, have reduced elasticity or extensibility, or contain contracted scar tissue. The main reason for the development of dysfunctional changes is the absence of adequate movement while contracture of soft tissues is occurring.

The age of the patient is usually above 30 years of age unless there is a preceding trauma or derangement. Posture is poor and a patient does not have a routine exercise program. So the onset can be sudden in case of trauma or otherwise it is a gradual onset pain. Dysfunction pain is experienced intermittently occurring only when the shortened structures are placed on full stretch, which is patient's end range. At this point, the shortened soft tissues are mechanically deformed. Pain is felt at the end range and never during the movement. With the exception of adherent neural tissue, pain from dysfunction is never referred into the arm or leg. When the end range stress is released, the pain decreases and disappears, only to return when the end range stress is applied again. The greater the loss of function the more often pain will occur. Pain results when patients engage in strenuous activity because they overstretch their adaptively shortened soft tissues causing microtrauma. Dysfunction as a result of poor posture or spondylosis tends to exhibit a symmetrical movement loss in all directions and many segments are involved. Dysfunction as a result of trauma or derangement more often has an asymmetrical movement loss.

Derangement Syndrome

Pain in the derangement syndrome arises as a result of disruption and or displacement within the intervertebral segment.

Postures involving unequal loading of the intervertebral disc causes the nucleus pulposus to become situated in an ever increasing eccentric position. This is of utmost importance in the development of discogenic discomfort and suggests its prevention. In the derangement syndrome, the normal resting position of articular surfaces of two adjacent vertebrae is disturbed as a result of this alteration in the position of nucleus between these surfaces. This leads to altered mechanical stress within and around the involved disc.

McKenzie stated that the main predisposing factors in the derangement syndrome is flexion, especially when sustained as in prolonged slouched sitting or stopped standing.

In flexion, the nucleus migrates posteriorly, the mechanical stress on the posterior structures of the spine is increased, and the disc pressure is increased compared to erect standing. In the lumbar spine, flexion especially combined flexion and rotation frequently lead to disc damage. There are two main types of derangement—posterior and anterior.

Posterior derangement is further divided into six different categories depending on the symptoms and extent of displacement of the nuclear annular complex. The posterior derangement is due to a posterior displacement of the nuclear/annular complex. It may also be associated with two acute deformities namely kyphosis and lateral shift deformity in the lumbar region or torticollis in cervical region.

In kyphosis there is flattening of the lumbar or cervical lordosis. Patient is not able to reverse this flattening on initial examination. The displacement of nucleus/annular complex obstructs the curve reversal and patient is locked in flexion. Lateral shift deformity is commonly referred to as list in lumbar region, acute torticollis or wryneck in cervical region. Cause for this is posterolateral derangement. The disc material has moved so far posterolaterally that the patient has to adopt this position so as to accommodate the deformity.

ANTERIOR DERANGEMENT

This is due to the antero or anterolateral migration of the nuclear /annular complex. Frequency of occurrence of anterior derangements is less as that of posterior derangement due to the fact that the anterior annulus is covered by the strong annular longitudinal ligament and that our flexion lifestyle places more stress on the posterior spinal structures. Patients with anterior derangement may present with a deformity of acute lumbar lordosis where flexion is blocked.

Clinical Picture

Derangement syndrome is commonly seen in age range of 20–55 years in the lumbar spine and 12–55 years in cervical region. Commonly, the onset of pain occurs during the first few hours of the day in the morning. Pain from derangement may alter its location and intensity. It may move proximally or distally or it may intensify or may diminish. When there is a change in location of the referred pain it may indicate that the intervertebral disc is changing its position. This occurs with movement or static positioning. Usually, there is no position in which the patient finds relief. Patients with posterior derangement in the lumbar spine often complain of increased pain during prolonged sitting or getting up from rising to sitting. Pain is usually less while standing walking or prone lying. This may be due to the fact that these activities allow anterior migration of the nucleus and thus reduce the derangement. Symptoms in cervical posterior derangements are also increased in activities involving flexion such as slouched sitting or looking down and are better when upright.

Management: McKenzie defines centralization as the phenomenon whereby as a result of the performance of certain repeated movements or the adoption of certain positions, radiating symptoms originating from the spine and referred distally are caused to move proximally towards the midline of the spine.

Movements that cause this phenomenon once identified can be used to abolish radiating or referred symptoms.

Where patients have pain of recent origin, this process can be extremely rapid and can in many cases occur in few minutes. The centralization of pain occurs only in derangement syndrome during the reductive process. As centralization takes place, there may be a significant increase of localized central pain adjacent to or in the spine itself.

Progression of forces: McKenzie's method is described as a progression of mechanical forces from patient to therapist generated. Following is an order of progression of forces which should be utilized by the therapist.

1. Static generated forces. Positioning in mid-range and in end range.
2. Dynamic patient generated forces: Patient motion in mid-range, patient motion in end range, patient motion in end range with overpressure.
3. Therapist generated forces: Patient motion to end range with therapist overpressure, therapist overpressure, mobilization/manipulation. Traction – Manual, intermittent or static.

Mobilization is defined as large amplitude, low velocity rhythmical passive movement up to the end of the available range of motion.

Manipulation—small amplitude high velocity single thrust passive movement at the end of available range of motion.

Traffic light principle: It can be used very effectively in any mechanical syndrome. To start with self-generated by the patient, progress to therapist generated. Only one technique can be added per session.

a. *Red light:* Pain is produce or increased and remains worsened (but not centralized).

   Inference:

   1. Direction of movement is incorrect and it increases the apparent disc displacement.
   2. Too rapid a movement to allow the reductive movement of the fluid nucleus/annulus complex.
   3. Dysfunction syndrome: Over forceful movement causes microtrauma.

b. *Amber light:* Derangement—pain that is produced or increased is not worsened.

   Pain that is decreased or abolished is not better as a result.

   Inference: Applied mechanical forces are not sufficient to produce a lasting change in the patients' symptoms.

c. *Green light:* Derangement—pain is decreased or abolished and remains better (centralized).

   Dysfunction: Pain produced at the end range disappears when the stretch is released.

   Inference: movement and degree of force is correct.

Management According to Syndromes

Postural syndrome: Once poor posture has been identified as the source of pain the treatment is geared towards postural correction. This requires close cooperation between patient and therapist. It is necessary for the patient to understand the fact that by continuing to adopt positions at end of range they are exposing their supporting structures to painful stimuli which they themselves can remove. For this patient can be put into the provocating posture, until the pain appears. Then by the simple act of correcting the posture patient is able to feel that the pain can be reduced by volition. Regular performance of such exercises will enable the patients to regain their postural awareness, moving from slouched posture to the erect posture. Use of the lumbar support in the correct way to maintain 90% of the position as passively as possible (Fig. 11.1).

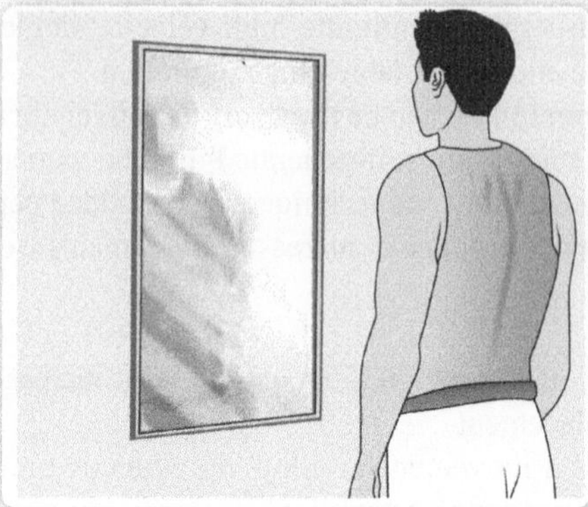

Fig. 11.1: Posture correction in front of posture mirror

Dysfunction Syndrome

Patients with dysfunction syndrome should be instructed about postural correction as removal of simple mechanical stresses may play an important role in the symptom correction. Also to achieve the desired tissue response, stretching procedures at the end of available range are ideally performed in a slow repeated movement fashion in sets of 10–15 every 2 hours throughout each day. In the treatment of dysfunction syndrome, manual procedures are introduced when progress is slow or nonexistent. The traffic light principle is still borne in mind to identify overstretching which may be causing trauma to the shortened structures. The use of rhythmical end of range mobilizations may also assist in lengthening of soft tissues but it should not replace the exercise program in any way (Fig. 11.2).

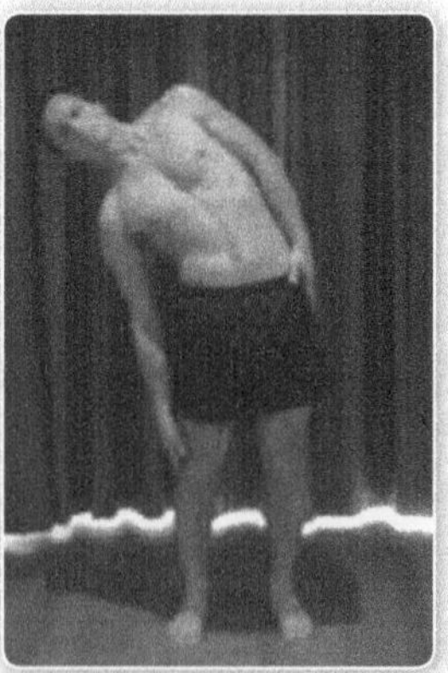

Fig. 11.2: Stretching of lateral trunk flexors

Derangement Syndrome

Reduction of the derangement: It is nothing but repositioning of the displaced material that is obstructing the spinal curve reversal or even forcing deformity. The diagnosis helps determine the appropriate direction of force required. The therapist should constantly be looking for positions and/or movements that centralize stop or decrease the pain, with centralization being the most important guide with the traffic light principal in action (Fig. 11.3).

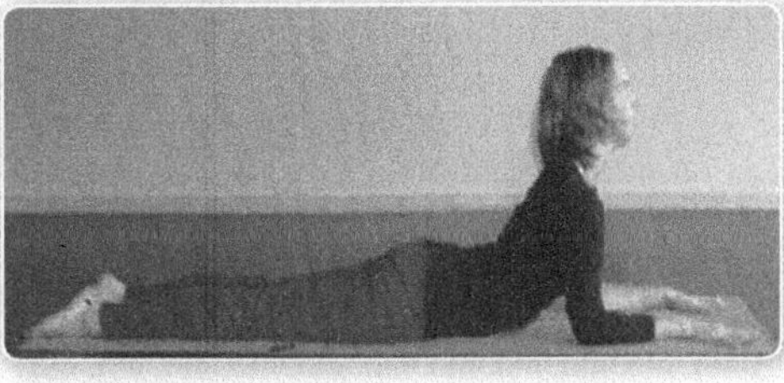

Fig. 11.3: Reduction of the derangement.

Maintenance of reduction: Just as a skin wound will reopen if the pulled on before it has healed sufficiently, so it seems that the reduced, derangement will recur if stressed too soon. For the posterior derangements it means that the patient must avoid both static and dynamic flexion and for the anterior derangement, extension. All derangement patients bar the lumbar anterior derangement must be educated in the maintenance of the axial extension posture.

During this time of maintenance of reduction, patient should continue his self-treatment program of appropriate exercises with addition of necessary exercises. The rules to observe the selection procedures are according to the mechanical diagnosis, progression of forces, centralization and traffic light guides.

Recovery of function: For this a gentle tension needs to be put on healing structures thus preventing future dysfunction. When the patient has complained of little or no pain for 2–3 days in the thoracolumbar spine and 24 hours in the cervical spine, then it is the time to introduce flexion movement. But testing needs to be carried out in the least forceful manner before introducing the flexion. So, if the patient experiences pain during the movement , increasing or peripheralizing the symptoms or remains worse following movement , then flexion is not yet safe to introduce as the derangement has not become stable.

Recovery of function is complete when full normal weight bearing flexion produces no more than the expected strain at the end of range.

Prophylaxis

Derangement can be prevented if the movement or static force is applied before displacement has a chance to recur. Once pain has returned or when the curve reversals are not possible or when the obstruction to curve reversals are emerging then the treatment not prevention is needed.

BIBLIOGRAPHY

1. Iebenson C. Rehabilitation of the spine: a practitioner's manual, second edition. Lipincott Williams and amp; Wilkins, Philadelphia 2007.
2. May S, Ross J et al. The McKenzie classification system in the extremities: A reliability study using McKenzie assessment forms and experienced clinicians. J manipul physiolog therapeut. 2009 Sep; 32 (7): 556-563.
3. McKenzie R., The lumbar spine: Mechanical diagnosis and therapy. Spinal publications. New-Zealand. 1981.

CHAPTER

12

Vojta Therapy

Learning Objectives

At the end of the chapter the learner shall be able to:

1. Describe the basic principles of Vojta therapy.
2. Define global patterns and explain its use in the treatment.
3. Describe the therapeutic goals.
4. Describe its use in various conditions.
5. Describe its effect on patient as a whole.
6. Enumerate contraindications.
7. Prescribe the therapy with appropriate duration.

INTRODUCTION

The Vojta principle was developed between 1950 and 1970 by the child neurologist Dr. Vaclav Vojta. It is also called as Reflex locomotion. It is a highly specialized type of physical therapy that is designed to primarily enhance the motor development of a child. Besides locomotion this therapy has added benefits of improvements in cognition, fine motor, breathing, and digestion.

"Global patterns" form the basis of reflex locomotion. These were discovered by Vojta in 1954. The term "global patterns" refers to the motor responses that arise during the application of reflex locomotion. Thus skeletal musculature throughout the entire body is activated in a coordinated manner and the central nervous system is addressed at all its regulatory levels.

The therapeutic goals of Reflex locomotion are:

1. To facilitate the automatic regulation or control of the body's position.

2. To facilitate the active maintenance of the support function of the extremities, and
3. To stimulate coordinated muscle activity.

These fundamental skills are disturbed to a greater or lesser extent in children with central or peripheral lesion of the nervous systems or impairment of the movement apparatus. This results in the pathological or substitute patterns of movement. These can be treated by reflex locomotion. In the Vojta method, normal patterns of movement sequences, for example, reaching and grasping, standing up and walking, are not taught or trained as such. Vojta therapy rather stimulates the brain, activating "innate, stored movement patterns" that are then "exported" as coordinated movements involving the musculature of the trunk and extremities. Vojta therapy has a positive influence on the entire coordination of a child in its spontaneous movement, resulting in improved up righting against gravity, balance, gait, grasp, speech and other functions. The improved coordination of movements as a result of the therapeutic "activation" can often be sustained over the duration of the whole day.

This therapy form, founded on the reflex locomotion, seeks to achieve the following:

- Alter the reflex activity of the child at rest as well as during the movements. This will lead to orientation of the neuromotor development towards a more physiological track. This is done by introducing a different central neurological activity that gives a fresh physical awareness to the patient. Muscular 'proprioception' plays an important role in this program.
- Alter the spinal automatisms in lesions of the spinal cord.
- Control breathing in order to increase basic parameters of respiration measured with the help of vital capacity.
- Control the neuro-vegetative reactions and promote balanced growth of the anatomical locomotor system.
- Prevent orthopedic complications which may hamper the progress of the child. It is so commonly seen in severe pathological conditions.

For example: Reflex creeping in a prone lying position and **reflex rolling** from a supine and side-lying position. Reflex creeping leads to a type of creeping movement, while reflex rolling begins from a supine lying position, and transforms, via a side-lying position, into the so-called quadruped gait.

In reflex locomotion, there is a coordinated, rhythmic activation of the total skeletal musculature and a CNS response at various circuit levels. The motor reactions, stimulated by pressure from a defined starting position and which proceed regularly and cyclically, can already be completely stimulated and reproduced as often as desired in the newborn.

All motor movements that appear in us in the development of grasping, rolling, crawling, standing up and walking are therefore activated visibly. They are – according to Prof Vojta – also already present in children, in a stage of development, in that children do not yet possess these abilities spontaneously.

Through therapeutic use of reflex locomotion, the – involuntary – muscle functions necessary for spontaneous movements in everyday life are activated in the patient, particularly in the spine, but also in the arms and legs, the hands and feet, as well as in the face.

Prof Vojta assumed that repeatedly stimulating these "reflex-like" movements lead to something like "freeing a switch" or "new networking" within functionally blocked networks of nerves between the patient's brain and spinal cord.

Goal of the Therapeutic Use of Reflex Locomotion

Through the use of the reflex locomotion, the elementary components of man's uprighting and locomotion, i.e.

- Equilibrium of the body when moving (postural regulation)
- Uprighting of the body against gravity
- Goal-directed grasping and stepping movements of the limbs (phasic mobility) should become accessible and usable once more.

The Difference from Other Physiotherapy Techniques and Methods

In Vojta Therapy movement functions, such as grasping, rolling over from the back onto the stomach or walking, are not practised. Rather, the therapeutic activation of reflex locomotion facilitates access, via the central nervous system, to the individual segmental patterns of movement necessary for a specific movement or activity.

After Vojta treatment, these segmental patterns are more available spontaneously to the patient. Regular repetition of the "normal movement" stored in the brain prevents evasion movements being practised. In any case, these would only be a substitute for the actual, and therefore desired, "normal movement".

Activating Vegetative and Other Automatic Reactions

With reflex locomotion, along with the “major” motor processes, also specific reactions such as:

- Conjugate eye movement (oculomotor activity)
- Tongue movements, jaw movements (orofacial motor activity).

As well as vegetative functions such as:

- Regulation of bladder and bowel function
- Breathing
- Sucking and swallowing can be activated and manipulated.

Reflex Locomotion and its Relation to Normal Motor Development

In all, the segmental patterns of reflex locomotion include all the building blocks of human motor development up to walking unaided. Through regular Vojta Therapy, the segmental patterns are “activated” in the central nervous system so that the activated state persists beyond the therapy, and the child/adult’s spontaneous movements are positively influenced.

According to clinical experience, a patient (child/adult) has a much more comprehensive—even normal—body posture after activation through reflex locomotion. This also gives the patient increasing emotional security to cope with the world around him and to build-up experience.

Application of Vojta Therapy in Children

Best results are obtained when the patient has not yet developed and established any so-called substitute motor patterns. In patients with established “substitute motor activity”, the goal of treatment is to activate and maintain physiological patterns of movement, as well as to reduce non-established abnormal patterns of movement and to integrate them into normal motor processes, all the way to complete mastery of conscious motor activity.

Application of Vojta Therapy in Newborn Babies

Vojta Therapy can equally be used in newborn babies as in children. It is indicated on the basis of a medical diagnosis and the accordingly formulated therapy goal.

The therapeutically desired activated state often expresses itself during treatment in newborn babies as crying. This understandably leads to parents feeling concerned, and makes them assume that it is "hurting" their child. At this age, however, crying is an important and appropriate means of expression for the little patients, who react in this way to unaccustomed activation. As a rule, after a short familiarization period, the crying is no longer so intense, and in breaks from exercise as well as after the therapy, newborn babies calm down immediately. In older children who can express themselves in speech, crying no longer occurs.

Effects of Vojta Therapy on Patient Development and Communication

With Vojta Therapy, there is the positive change in movement coordination in grasping, uprighting against gravity, walking and speaking. As a consequence of this change, the child or adult is afterwards able to express his wishes and needs more easily and comprehensively and to fulfill them spontaneously. Patients are less frustrated, and seem happier and more balanced. Older children or adults say that after Vojta treatment they feel "lighter" when they move. Such a positive emotional basis leads to a visibly improved ability to communicate. Overall, Vojta Therapy gives the patient significantly improved possibilities for motor learning as he negotiates the world around him.

Aside from Vojta Therapy, no constant observation or corrective intervention by the parents is necessary, so the newborn baby or child can move freely and spontaneously. According to the Vojta Principle, there are no incorrect postures that could hinder the success of the treatment.

Because Vojta Therapy "activates" postural and movement functions in the newborn baby or child's central nervous system, the improved level of movement that they reach in the required few and short daily therapy units can, as a rule, be maintained over the whole day.

As a result, this also encourages the little patient to develop self-reliance and independence from adults. This is a desired goal of the treatment. Vojta Therapy likewise encourages parents in their parental role: In daily Vojta Therapy, the child experiences physical contact and a parental guidance that conveys security. Vojta Therapy thus strengthens the parent-child relationship and leads to new, enhanced experiences for the child.

Contraindications for Vojta Therapy

Vojta Therapy should not be used in:

- Acute feverish or inflammatory conditions
- Vaccinations with live vaccines following doctor's orders (as a rule 10 days after vaccination)
- Existing pregnancy in patients
- Certain illness, as e.g. imperfect osteogenesis, heart disease, etc.

In all illnesses that impact on patient's general condition, Vojta Therapy can be carried out for shorter sessions, depending on the tolerance level of the patient, but does not have to be ruled out.

General Issues in Relation to the Treatment with Vojta Therapy

Parents/Caregivers

Since parents or caregivers perform the therapy several times a day, they play a decisive role in Vojta Therapy.

In the treatment of adult patients, Vojta Therapy can be performed by a spouse, life partner or someone close. In this instance, therapy is, as a rule, performed several times a week.

Instruction and Performance of Vojta Therapy

As well as the primary illness, exercise intensity and accuracy determine the effectiveness and ultimately the success of the Vojta treatment. After referral to Vojta Therapy by the doctor, the Vojta therapist draws up an individual program and determines the goals of therapy jointly with the patient/parents. The therapy program is then determined at regular intervals in accordance with the patient's development.

For Vojta therapy to be successful, it must be carried out several times a day. A treatment lasts between 5–20 minutes. Because the parents carry out the treatment daily, they play a very important role in the implementation of Vojta therapy.

For the entire duration of the therapy—which can last for weeks to months, or years—the Vojta therapist educates the parents how to implement the therapy and is a support person for the parents. The therapy program, the amount, the pauses from therapy, etc. is regularly reviewed in relationship to the patient's progress and development.

BIBLIOGRAPHY

1. Vojta V. The basic elements of treatment according to Vojta. In: Scrutton D, (Ed). Management of the Motor Disorders of Children with Cerebral Palsy. Oxford: Spastics Int Med. Public. Blackwell Sc. Public. Ltd. 1984: 75-85.
2. Kanda T, Yuge M, Yamori Y et al. Early physiotherapy in the treatment of spastic diplegia. Dev Med Child Neurol. 1984; 26: 438-44.
3. Imamura S, Sakuma K, Takahashi T. Follow-up study of children with Ccrcbral Coordination Disturbancc (CCD): (a) Int. Congress of Child Neurology, Tokyo. 1980; (b) Brain Dev. 1983; 5: 311-4.

CHAPTER

13

Constraint-induced Movement Therapy

Learning Objectives

At the end of the topic the learner shall be able to:

1. Describe basic concept of CIMT.
2. Describe inclusion criteria for CIMT.
3. Describe methodology used in the treatment technique.

Constraint-induced movement therapy (CIMT) or forced use is a technique designed to promote increased use of weak or paralyzed arm and has been credited with speeding up the cortical map reorganization process in nonhuman primates and in humans. It is also based on principles of dynamic systems theory and task oriented approach to motor control acquisition. In other methods of stroke rehabilitation, clients learn to use the stronger, or less involved arm for daily activities. This type of treatment approach may foster learned nonuse of the stronger arm.

Learned nonuse is proposed to be a phenomenon in which individual effectively forgets to use the affected or involved extremity because of the extreme difficulty coordinating movement after the onset of a stroke. Animal research has led to the discovery that cortical reorganization occurs after injury to the nervous system. Taub theorized that use of differenced extremity can be regained if the intact extremity is restrained and the monkey is forced to use the extremity. If the restraint was used to for a specific period of time between 1 to 2 weeks, return of function could be permanent.

Another technique, shaping, has also shown substantial improvements in motor function in daily life situations. Shaping procedures are behavioral techniques that approach a desired motor outcome in small, successive increments. Shaping techniques allow subjects to experience successful gains in performance with relatively small amounts of motor improvement. CIT forces clients to use the affected upper extremity in a sling mitt, or a combination of both. Clients then practice using their affected extremity on an intensive basis for several consecutive weeks by using shaping movements with the weaker arm. Taub described this phenomenon as learned nonuse, thus part of the theoritical framework of CIT is taken from the neurophysiological and behavioral studies of learned nonuse of the weaker limb seen in animal experimentation.

Typically the inclusion criteria for CIT is a first time CVA that occurred more than a year ago.

- Not currently receiving therapeutic intervention;
- A score of $\geq$ 44 on BBS or limited balance problems requiring an assistive device for mobility in clients who had a full time care giver to assist with any balance issues;
- Ability to move the affected arm in 45 degrees shoulder flexion and abduction, 90° elbow flexion and extension, 20° wrist extension and 10° extension at metacarpal phalanges and interphalanges as determined by active ROM;
- No significant cognitive deficits as demonstrated by MMS score of at least 22;
- No pre-existing co morbidities that might interfere with mobility or function;
- Limited spasticity as measured on MAS;
- Ability to identify an individual to assist with the home program.

In summary, potential reasons for a person to be excluded may include motor ability that is too high or too low, cognitive deficits that prevent adequate participation and an already high use of the weaker arm.

Therapeutic procedures using CIMT in the clinic are performed under supervision from the therapist. The procedures are effective only if the use of the weaker arm is carried over in the home environment. Clients are asked about their compliance in filling out a daily entry in their home diaries. Home diary is used to outline the client's activities from the time at which they are discharged from the clinic until they return for their daily sessions. A typical daily schedule is often used.

In brief CI therapy involves 3 main elements: (1) Intensive training of the more affected arm (2) A transfer package of techniques to promote transfer of therapeutic gains from laboratories to the real world environment (3) Motor restriction of the less affected arm during the entire period of treatment.

The ratio of therapist to client is typically 1:1. Therapist is expected to give tactile and verbal feedback for the tasks assigned. Also therapist should encourage and if needed, assist the patient to complete the task. To perform the task, the unaffected arm is kept in a sling or glove for almost 90% of the waking hours for 2–3 weeks. During this time, patient is also given a concentrated, repetitive task training of the more affected arm using functional activities of daily living. Tasks trained during CIMT can be divided into two broad categories: rote generic tasks, such as grasping puzzle pieces, marbles, or cones, and functional occupation-based tasks that are meaningful and purposeful for the patient.

Research is also done with modification of CIMT using mental practice as an adjunct. Wherein, it was found that modified constraint-induced therapy again rendered clinically significant changes. However, data also suggest that the addition of MP to the mCIT protocol renders comparatively larger motor changes than mCIT participation alone.

The application of CIMT to real life clinical environments presents some challenges including the time and physical demands on therapists and resources of rehabilitation unit limiting its cost effectiveness and overall effect. The future success of CIMT will depend on its ability to be modified according to the disease factors economic considerations, limitations of practice setting, and the cognitive and physical status of the patient.

BIBLIOGRAPHY

1. Taub E, Miller NE, Novack TA, Cook EW, Fleming WC, Nepomuceno CS, et al. Technique to improve chronic motor deficit after stroke. Arch Phys Med Rehabil. 1993;74:347–54.
2. Umphred DM, Neurological Rehabilitiaion, 5th edn. Mosby Elsevier Publication. 2007.
3. Van der Lee JH, Wagenaar RC, Lankhorst GJ, Vogelaar TW, Devillé WL, Bouter LM. Forced use of the upper extremity in chronic stroke patients: results from a single-blind randomized clinical trial. Stroke. 1999;30:2369–75.
4. Stephen J, Peter Levine, Khoury JC. Modified Constraint-induced Therapy Combined With Mental Practice, Stroke. 2009;40:551.

CHAPTER

14

TheraTogs

Learning Objectives

At the end of the chapter learner shall be able to:

1. Describe the basic principles of TheraTogs.
2. Describe the components of TheraTogs.
3. Describe the basic application.

It is an orthotic undergarment fabricated from Delta-flex, a light weighted, breathable fabric that is Velcro sensitive. It has been developed to provide a gentle passive force to correct imbalance or alignment through a combination of trunk and short systems along with a customized external strapping system. It can improve joint stability, posture and gait skills. It provides vertical stiffness to reinforce postural stability, and horizontal stretch for mild compression and a comfortable fit. A TheraTogs garment consists of a tank top and shorts that are designed to be worn directly on the skin. TheraTogs are made from a patented, proprietary, machine-washable composite fabric consisting of nylon and spandex with an inner foam layer that gently grips the skin and the underlying soft tissues, and a Velcrosensitive outer layer to which your therapist can affix elastic strapping, to effectively influence your child's movement, stability, posture and gait. It provides access for toileting when the system is worn during the day, improving the ease of wear. This system is an exomuscular system that the patient will eventually wear almost 16 hours a day. They are made from an inner layer and adjustable Velcro straps. It provides deep pressure sensory input, increase attention and improves body awareness. The gentle compression increases neurosensory feedback for planning movements. Children with low or high muscle tone benefit from strapping that attaches to the Velcro sensitive material to reinforce postural alignment and efficient use of muscles.

Principles: It works by applying consistent, gentle compression and proprioceptive input to the skin and underlying muscles and joints to facilitate the activation of those muscles.

Addition of straps to the basic TheraTogs garment will assist weak underused muscles reducing postural convexities and realigning functional muscles and joints.

The TheraTogs sensory integration system is designed to help children, who have difficulty with issues such as hypersensitivity, focusing attention, stimming, sitting still, and coordinating movement. TheraTogs are especially effective at calming patient Alibrss and increasing student attention—which can help improve the practice and efficacy of other management modalities.

The TheraTogs sensory integration (SI) system applies gentle, consistent vertical compression through the torso and lateral compression through the hip joints to provide calming proprioceptive, tactile, and deep pressure input that has been shown to help some children with SI dysfunction or sensory processing issues to regain body awareness, postural stability, attention, coordination, breath volume and control, and balance. This type of compression is more specific, more dynamic, and more variable than a cumbersome weighted vest. TheraTogs give a 'wearable hug' that is worn discreetly under clothing.

One of the key benefits of TheraTogs is carry-over between therapy sessions. The therapist can send children home from a successful therapy session with a TheraTogs system that continues to deliver gains made in postural alignment, muscle function, and sensory processing. Rather than receive only 1 to 3 hours of therapy per week.

THERATOGS AND BIOMECHANICAL DIFFICULTIES

TheraTogs apply prolonged, low-load (gentle) forces to the musculoskeletal system to effect changes in muscle recruitment strategies, and, with full-time use, in muscle physiology and bone geometry.

To gain optimum posture and function, thousands or repetitions of movements must occur in optimum alignment. TheraTogs accomplishes this by wrapping the torso in a Velcro-sensitive garment that serves as a 'strapping field,' allowing the therapist to attach straps that work like external muscles to improve postural alignment and stability and potentially address a wide variety of functional alignment and movement issues. The therapist will mark the TheraTogs garment for correct positioning of the TheraTogs straps, and instruct the parent in how to put them on their child.

SPECIFIC EXAMPLES

Poor Postural Alignment

Correct postural alignment consists of the spine being positioned in the most efficient way, so that the body does not waste energy in keeping the head upright, and the bones are not at risk of rubbing together in a manner that will cause damage to the joints. Poor postural alignment can be caused by weak abdominal muscles, resulting in an excessive curve in the lower back. The therapist would design the TheraTogs strapping to facilitate activation of the abdominal muscles to help strengthen the muscles and to assist in proper alignment of the spine to reduce the excessive curve in the lower back.

Cerebral Palsy

A child with cerebral palsy often has difficulty walking because the high muscle tone, or spasticity, often causes the legs to cross as the child walks. The therapist would design, and then demonstrate to the parent, a strapping system to help the weaker muscles work more effectively to pull the leg straight as the child steps forward.

TheraTogs have been shown to be effective in addressing issues in diagnoses that result in sensory processing difficulties or biomechanical problems such as: sensory processing disorder, autism spectrum disorder, attention deficit disorders, coordination deficits, balance deficits hypotonia.

Cerebral palsy ataxia, intoed gait, out-toed gait, mild weakness, flexible joint, deviations, muscle recruitment problems, pain due to muscle imbalances, joint laxity, postural malalignment.

Use TheraTogs to

- Promote optimum bone and joint development
- Provide joint stability and increased body awareness
- Improve posture, balance, gait, and movement skills
- Reduce the postural correction workload that is often expected of foot and ankle orthoses
- Improve motor performance during therapy sessions

- "Send the therapist's hands home" in support of the therapy program between sessions
- Custom fit each client with a cozy, non-slip TheraTogs™ set and an elastic strapping and support system designed to address that client's specific musculoskeletal, postural, balance, or movement issues. Select from a variety of strap designs, lengths, widths, alibris of stiffness and placement options to optimize their therapeutic and orthotic influences.

BIBLIOGRAPHY

1. Abel MF, Damiano DL, Blanco JS, et al. Relationships among musculoskeletal impairments and functional health status in ambulatory cerebral palsy. J Pediatr Orthop. 2003; 23(4): 535-541.
2. Adolph KE, Vereijken B, Shrout PE. What changes in infant walking and why. Child Dev. 2003; 74(2):475-97.
3. Adolph KE. Learning in the development of infant locomotion. Monogr Soc Res Child Dev. 1997; 62(3):I-VI, 1-158.
4. Fisher B. Effect of trunk control and alignment on limb function. J Head Trauma Rehabil. 1987; 2(2):72.

APPENDICES

Appendix I

National Institute of Health Stroke Scale

1A: Level of Consciousness

(If intubated, make best guess, but only choose 3 if posturing/unresponsive)

- Alert; keenly responsive 0
- Not alert, but arousable by minor stimulation 1
- Not alert, requires repeated stimulation to arouse 2
- Not alert/obtunded, makes movements to pain 3
- Postures or unresponsive to pain 4.

1B: Ask Month and Age

- Answers both questions correctly 0
- Answers one question correctely 1
- Answers neither questions right 2
- Aphasic UN

1C: Tell patient to Open and Close Eyes, then Hand Grip Squeeze (Substitute/Pantomime Commands if Language Barrier/Confusion)

- Performs both tasks correctly 0
- Performs one task correctly 1
- Performs 0 tasks correctly 2

2: Test Horizontal Extraocular Movements

- Normal: Able to move both eyes left to right across midline 0
- Partial gaze palsy: Gaze is abnormal in one or both eyes, but forced deviation, or total gaze paresis is not present. Able to move one or both eyes, but may not be able to cross midline 1
- Forced deviation: Total gaze paresis is not overcome by the oculocephalic maneuver 2

3. Visual Field

- No visual loss 0
- Partial hemianopia: Includes loss in only one quadrant 1

- Complete hemianopia: Loss of vision in both top and bottom quadrants on the right or left side 2
- Bilateral hemianopia: Blindness of any cause, or if visual loss is noted on both right and left sides 3

4: Test Facial Palsy

(Use Grimace if Obtunded)

- Normal: Symmetrical movements 0
- Minor paralysis: Flattened nasolabial fold, asymmetry on smiling 1
- Partial paralysis: Total or near-total paralysis of lower face 2
- Complete paralysis of one or both sides of face 3

5A: Test Left Arm Motor Drift

- No drift, limb holds 90° (or 45°) for a full 10 seconds 0
- Drift, limb holds 90° (or 45°), but then drifts down before full 10 seconds; does not hit bed 1
- Some effort against gravity, limb cannot get to or maintain 90° (or 45°), drifts down to bed, but has some effort against gravity 2
- No effort against gravity: Limb fall 3
- No movement, flaccid extremities with no effort noted 4
- Amputation/joint fusion UN

5B: Test Right Arm Motor Drift

- No drift, limb holds 90° (or 45°) for a full 10 seconds 0
- Drift, limb holds 90° (or 45°), but then drifts down before full 10 seconds; does not hit bed 1
- Some effort against gravity, limb cannot get to or maintain 90° (or 45°), drifts down to bed, but has some effort against gravity 2
- No effort against gravity: Limb fall 3
- No movement, flaccid extremities with no effort noted 4
- Amputation/joint fusion UN

6A: Test Left Leg Motor Drift

- No drift leg holds 30° position for full five seconds 0
- Drift, leg falls by the end of the five second period but does not hit bed 1
- Some effort against gravity: Leg falls to bed by five seconds, but has some effort against gravity 2
- No effort against gravity: Leg falls to bed immediately 3
- No movement: Flaccid extremities with no effort noted

6B: Test Right Leg Motor Drift

- No drift leg holds 30° position for full five seconds 0
- Drift, leg falls by the end of the five second period but does not hit bed 1
- Some effort against gravity: Leg falls to bed by five seconds, but has some effort against gravity 2
- No effort against gravity: Leg falls to bed immediately 3
- No movement: Flaccid extremities with no effort noted 4

7. Test Limb Ataxia (FNF/Heel-Shin)

- No ataxia 0
- Ataxia in 1 limb 1
- Ataxia in 2 limbs 2
- Paralyzed 3
- Amputation/joint fusion UN

8: Test Sensation

- Normal: No sensory loss 0
- Mild-moderate loss: Can sense being touched 1
- Complete loss: Cannot sense being touched at all 2
- Coma/unresponsive UN

9: Test Language/Aphasia

(Describe the scene; name the words; read the sentences.)

- Normal: No aphasia 0
- Mild-moderate aphasia: Some obvious changes, without significant limitation 1
- Severe aphasia: Fragmentary expression, inference needed, cannot identify materials 2
- Mute/global aphasia: No usable speech/auditory comprehension 3

10: Test Dysarthria

(Read the words)

- Normal 0
- Mild-moderate dysarthria: Slurring but can be understood 1
- Severe dysarthria: Unintelligble slurring or out of proportion to dysphasia 2
- Intubated/unable to test UN

11: Test Extinction/Inattention

- No abnormality 0
- Visual, tactile, auditory, special or personal inattention or extinction to bilateral simultaneous stimulation in one of the sensory modalities 1

- Profound hemi-inattention: Patient does not recognize own hand or orients to only one side of space 2

Interpretation: Total Score is Out of 42

- 0–No stroke symptoms
- 1–4—Minor stroke
- 5–15—Moderate stroke
- 16–20—Moderate to severe stroke
- 21–42—Severe stroke

BIBLIOGRAPHY

1. Kasner SE, Chalela JA, Luciano JM, Cucchiara BL, Raps EC, McGarvey ML, et al. Reliability and validity of estimating the NIH Stroke Scale score from medical records. Stroke. 1999;30:1534-7.
2. Williams LS, Yilmaz EY, Lopez-Yunez AM. Retrospective assessment of initial stroke severity with the NIH Stroke Scale. Stroke. 2000;31:858-62.

Appendix II

Canadian Neurological Scale

1. **Level of Consciousness**
   - Alert: 3.0 points
   - Drowsy: 1.5 points
2. **Orientation (Ask month in year)**
   - Oriented: 1 points
   - Disoriented, not applicable: 0 points
3. **Speech**
   - (Ask 1. To close eye. 2. Point to ceiling. 3. Does a stone sink in water), if does not complete the above 3, go to section A2)
   - Receptive deficit: 0.0 point
   - Expressive deficit: 0.5 point
   - Normal speech: 0 points

SECTION A1: NO COMPREHENSION DEFICIT

1. **Face (Ask to Smile) :**
   - No facial weakness: 0.5 point
   - Facial weakness presents: 0 points
2. **Proximal Arm** (Ask to lift arm to shoulder level, apply resistance above elbow)
   - No weakness : 1.5 points
   - Mild weakness : 1 point (Movement to 90°, unable to oppose pressure)
   - Significant weakness: 0.5 points (movement < 90°)
   - Paralysis: 0 points
3. **Distal Arm** (Ask to bend wrist back and apply pressure)
   - No weakness: 1.5 points
   - Mild weakness: 1 point (Can bend wrist, unable to oppose pressure)
   - Significant weakness: 0.5 points
   - Paralysis: 0 point (Absence of movement)

4. **Proximal Leg** (Ask to flex knee to 90°, push down on each thigh one at time)
    - No weakness: 1.5 points
    - Mild weakness: 1.0 point (Can lift leg, unable to oppose pressure)
    - Significant weakness: 0.5 points (Lateral movement but no power to lift leg)
    - Paralysis: 0 points (Absence of movement)
5. **Distal Leg** (Ask to point toes of feet upward. push down on each foot one at time)
    - No weakness 1.5 points
    - Mild weakness: 1 point (Can point upward, unable to oppose pressure)
    - Significant weakness: 0.5 points (Some movement at toes, but cannot lift toes)
    - Paralysis: 0 points

SECTION A2 COMPREHENSION DEFICIT

1. **Face** (Ask point to mimic your grin)
    - Symmetrical: 0.5 point
    - Asymmetrical: 0 point
2. **Arms**
    - (Place patient arm in front of point at 90° (If unable, apply finger nailed pressure bilaterally and compare response)
    - Equal: 1.5 points (Equal motor response)
    - Unequal: 0 points (Unequal motor response)
3. **Legs**
    - (Thigh flexed to 90°, if unable, apply to nail bed pressure bilaterally and compare response)
    - Equal: 1.5 points (Maintain position or withdraw equally)
    - Unequal: 0 points (Cannot maintain position)
    - Interpretation: Total score is out of 11.5
    - Score: 8—Mild Impairment
    - Score: 5–7—Moderate Impairment
    - Score: 1–4—Severe Impairment

BIBLIOGRAPHY

1. Cote R, Battista RN, Wolfson C, Boucher J, Adam J, Hachinski V. The Canadian Neurological Scale: validation and reliability assessment. Neurology. 1989;39:638-3.
2. Goldstein LB, Chilukuri V. Retrospective assessment of initial stroke severity with the Canadian Neurological Scale. Stroke. 1997;28:1181-4.

Appendix III

The Barthel Index

Patient Name: ____________________________

Rater Name: ____________________________

Date: ____________________________

Activity **Score**

Feeding

- 0 = Unable
- 5 = Needs help cutting, spreading butter, etc. or requires modified diet
- 10 = Independent ______

Bathing

- 0 = Dependent
- 5 = Independent (or in shower) ______

Grooming

- 0 = Needs to help with personal care
- 5 = Independent face/hair/teeth/shaving
  (implements provided) ______

Dressing

- 0 = Dependent
- 5 = Needs help but can do about half unaided
- 10 = Independent (including buttons, zips, laces, etc.) ______

Bowels

- 0 = Incontinent (or needs to be given enemas)
- 5 = Occasional accident
- 10 = Continent ______

Bladder

- 0 = Incontinent, or catheterized and unable to manage alone
- 5 = Occasional accident
- 10 = Continent ______

Toilet Use

- 0 = Dependent
- 5 = Needs some help, but can do something alone
- 10 = Independent (on and off, dressing, wiping) ______

Transfers (Bed to Chair and Back)

- 0 = Unable, no sitting balance
- 5 = Major help (one or two people, physical), can sit
- 10 = Minor help (verbal or physical)
- 15 = Independent ______

Mobility (On Level Surfaces)

- 0 = Immobile or < 50 yards
- 5 = Wheelchair independent, including corners, > 50 yards
- 10 = Walks with help of one person (verbal or physical) > 50 yards
- 15 = Independent (but may use any aid; for example, stick)

> 50 Yards ______

Stairs

- 0 = Unable
- 5 = Needs help (verbal, physical, carrying aid)
- 10 = independent ______
- Total (0–100): ______

THE BARTHEL ADL INDEX: GUIDELINES

1. The index should be used as a record of what a patient does, not as a record of what a patient could do.
2. The main aim is to establish degree of independence from any help, physical or verbal, however minor and for whatever reason.
3. The need for supervision renders the patient not independent.
4. A patient's performance should be established using the best available evidence. Asking the patient, friends/relatives and nurses are the usual sources, but direct observation and common sense are also important. However, direct testing is not needed.

5. Usually the patient's performance over the preceding 24–48 hours is important, but occasionally longer periods will be relevant.
6. Middle categories imply that the patient supplies over 50 percent of the effort.
7. Use of aids to be independent is allowed.

BIBLIOGRAPHY

1. Gresham GE, Phillips TF, Labi ML. "ADL status in stroke: relative merits of three standard indexes." Arch Phys Med Rehabil. 1980;61:355-8.
2. Loewen SC, Anderson BA. "Predictors of stroke outcome using objective measurement scales." Stroke. 1990;21:78-81.
3. Mahoney FI, Barthel D. "Functional evaluation: the Barthel Index." Maryland State Medical Journal. 1965;14:56-61.

Appendix IV

Functional Independence Measure

4. Roy CW, Togneri J, Hay E, Pentland B. An inter-rater reliability study of the Barthel Index. Int J Rehabil Res. 1988;11:67-70.

FUNCTIONAL INDEPENDENCE MEASURE

The Functional Independence Measure (FIM) scale assesses physical and cognitive disability. This scale focuses on the burden of care – that is, the level 1 of disability indicating the burden of caring for them.

Scoring

Items are scored on the level of assistance required for an individual to perform activities of daily living. The scale includes 18 items, of which 13 items are physical domains based on the Barthel Index and 5 items are cognition items.

Each item is scored from 1 to 7 based on level of independence, where 1 represents total dependence and 7 indicates complete independence. The scale can be administered by a physician, nurse, therapist or layperson. Possible scores range from 7 to 126, with higher scores indicating more independence.

Components

Self-care

1. Eating
2. Grooming
3. Bathing/showering

4. Dressing upper body
5. Dressing lower body
6. Toileting.

Sphincters

1. Bladder management.
2. Bowel management.

Mobility

1. Transfers: Bed/chair/wheelchair.
2. Transfers: Toilet.
3. Transfers: Bathtub/shower.
4. Locomotion: Walking/wheelchair.
5. Locomotion: Stairs.

Communication

1. Expression
2. Comprehension.

Psychosocial

1. Social interaction.

Cognition

1. Problem solving
2. Memory.

Seven Levels for Each Item

Level Description

7 Complete independence: Fully independent.
6 Modified independence: Requiring the use of a device but no physical help.
5 Supervision: Requiring only standby assistance or verbal prompting or help with set-up.
4 Minimal assistance: Requiring incidental hands-on help only (subject performs > 75% of the task).
3 Moderate assistance: Subject still performs 50–75% of the task.

2 Maximal assistance: Subject provides less than half of the effort (25–49%).
1 Total assistance: Subject contributes < 25% of the effort or is unable to do the task.

Scoring Principles

- Function is assessed on the basis of direct observation.
- Admission scoring is done within 10 days of admission.
- Discharge scoring is done during the last week before discharge.
- Scoring is done by a multi-disciplinary team member.

The subject is scored on what they actually do on a day-to-day basis, not on what they could do. Do not leave any score blank.

Score 1, if the subject does not perform the activity at all, or if no information is available. If function is variable, use the lower score.

BIBLIOGRAPHY

1. Hall KM, Mann N, High WM, *et al.* Functional measures after traumatic brain injury: ceiling effects of FIM, FIM+FAM, DRS and CIQ. J Head Trauma Rehabil. 1996;11: 27-39.
2. Hamilton BB, Granger CV, Sherwin FS, et al. A uniform national data system for medical rehabilitation. In: Fuhrer MJ, (ed). Rehabilitation Outcomes: analysis and measurement. Baltimore, MD: Brookes; 1987; pp.137–47.
3. Stineman MG, Jette A, Fiedler R, et al. Impairment-specifi c dimensions within the Functional Independence Measure. Arch Phys Med Rehabil. 1997; 78:636-43.
4. Turner-Stokes L, Nyein K, Turner-Stokes T, et al. The UK FIM+FAM: development and evaluation. Clin Rehabil. 1999;13:277-87.

Appendix V

Appendix. *STroke REhabilitation Assessment of Movement (STREAM)*[©]

Assessment Dates (Y/M/D)

1.
2.
3.
4.

Patient's Name: ____________________

Date of CVA: __________ **Sex:** M F **Age:** ______

Side of Lesion: L R **Side of Hemiplegia:** L R

Comorbid Conditions: ____________________

Type of aid(s) used: ____________________

Physiotherapist(s): ____________________

General Comments: ____________________

STREAM SCORING

I. VOLUNTARY MOVEMENT OF THE LIMBS

0 unable to perform the test movement through any appreciable range (includes flicker or slight movement)
1 a. able to perform only **part** of the movement, and with **marked deviation** from normal pattern
b. able to perform only **part** of the movement, but in a manner that is **comparable to the unaffected side**
c. able to **complete** the movement, but only with **marked deviation** from normal pattern
2 able to **complete** the movement in a manner that is **comparable to the unaffected side**
X activity not tested (specify why: ROM, Pain, Other (reason))

II. BASIC MOBILITY

0 unable to perform the test activity through any appreciable range (ie, minimal active participation)
1 a. able to perform only **part** of the activity independently (requires partial assistance or stabilization to complete), with or without an aid, and with **marked deviation** from normal pattern
b. able to perform only **part** of the activity independently (requires partial assistance or stabilization to complete), with or without an aid, but with a grossly **normal** movement pattern
c. able to **complete** the activity independently, with or without an aid, but only with **marked deviation** from normal pattern
2 able to **complete** the activity independently with a grossly **normal** movement pattern, but **requires an aid**
3 able to **complete** the activity independently with a grossly **normal** movement pattern, **without an aid**
X activity not tested (specify why: ROM, Pain, Other (reason))

		AMPLITUDE OF ACTIVE MOVEMENT		
		None	Partial	Complete
MOVEMENT QUALITY	Marked Deviation	0	1 a	1 c
	Grossly Normal	0	1 b	2 (3)

SCORE 4	3	2	1		
					SUPINE
				/2	1. PROTRACTS SCAPULA IN SUPINE *"Lift your shoulder blade so that your hand moves towards the ceiling"* **Note:** therapist stabilizes arm with shoulder 90° flexed and elbow extended.
				/2	2. EXTENDS ELBOW IN SUPINE (starting with elbow fully flexed) *"Lift your hand towards the ceiling, straightening your elbow as much as you can"* **Note:** therapist stabilizes arm with shoulder 90° flexed; strong associated shoulder extension and/or abduction=marked deviation (score 1a or 1c).
				/2	3. FLEXES HIP AND KNEE IN SUPINE (attains half crook lying) *"Bend your hip and knee so that your foot rests flat on the bed"*
				/3	4. ROLLS ONTO SIDE (starting from supine) *"Roll onto your side"* **Note:** may roll onto <u>either</u> side; pulling with arms to turn over=aid (score 2).
				/3	5. RAISES HIPS OFF BED IN CROOK LYING (BRIDGING) *"Lift your hips as high as you can"* **Note:** therapist may stabilize foot, but if knee pushes strongly into extension with bridging=marked deviation (score 1a or 1c); if requires aid (external or from therapist) to maintain knees in midline=aid (score 2).
				/3	6. MOVES FROM LYING SUPINE TO SITTING (with feet on the floor) *"Sit up and place your feet on the floor"* **Note:** may sit up to <u>either</u> side using any functional and safe method; longer than 20 seconds=marked deviation (score 1a or 1c); pulling up using bedrail or edge of plinth=aid (score 2).
					SITTING (feet supported; hands resting on pillow on lap for items 7-14)
				/2	7. SHRUGS SHOULDERS (SCAPULAR ELEVATION) *"Shrug your shoulders as high as you can"* **Note:** both shoulders are shrugged simultaneously.
				/2	8. RAISES HAND TO TOUCH TOP OF HEAD *"Raise your hand to touch the top of your head"*
				/2	9. PLACES HAND ON SACRUM *"Reach behind your back and as far across toward the other side as you can"*
				/2	10. RAISES ARM OVERHEAD TO FULLEST ELEVATION *"Reach your hand as high as you can towards the ceiling"*

SCORE 4	3	2	1		
				/2	11. **SUPINATES <u>AND</u> PRONATES FOREARM** (elbow flexed at 90°) *"Keeping your elbow bent and close to your side, turn your forearm over so that your palm faces up, then turn your forearm over so that your palm faces down"* **Note:** movement in one direction only=partial movement (score 1a or 1b).
				/2	12. **CLOSES HAND FROM FULLY OPENED POSITION** *"Make a fist, keeping your thumb on the outside"* **Note:** must extend wrist slightly (ie, wrist cocked) to obtain full marks; full fist with lack of wrist extention=partial movement (score 1a or 1b).
				/2	13. **OPENS HAND FROM FULLY CLOSED POSITION** *"Now open your hand all the way"*
				/2	14. **OPPOSES THUMB TO INDEX FINGER** (tip to tip) *"Make a circle with your thumb and index finger"*
				/2	15. **FLEXES HIP IN SITTING** *"Lift your knee as high as you can"*
				/2	16. **EXTENDS KNEE IN SITTING** *"Straighten your knee by lifting your foot up"*
				/2	17. **FLEXES KNEE IN SITTING** *"Slide your foot back under you as far as you can"* **Note:** start with affected foot forward (heel in line with toes of other foot).
				/2	18. **DORSIFLEXES ANKLE IN SITTING** *"Keep your heel on the ground and lift your toes off the floor as far as you can"* **Note:** affected foot is placed slightly forward (heel in line with toes of other foot).
				/2	19. **PLANTAR FLEXES ANKLE IN SITTING** *"Keep your toes on the ground and lift your heel off the floor as far as you can"*
				/2	20. **EXTENDS KNEE <u>AND</u> DORSIFLEXES ANKLE IN SITTING** *"Straighten your knee and bring your toes towards you"* **Note:** extension of knee without dorsiflexion of ankle=partial movement (score 1a or 1b).
				/3	21. **RISES TO STANDING FROM SITTING** *"Stand up; try to take equal weight on both legs"* **Note:** pushing up with hand(s) to stand=aid (score 2); asymmetry such as trunk lean, Trendelenburg position, hip retraction, or excessive flexion or extension of the affected knee=marked deviation (score 1a or 1c).

SCORE 4	3	2	1		
					STANDING
				/3	22. MAINTAINS STANDING FOR 20 COUNTS *"Stand on the spot while I count to twenty"*
					STANDING (holding onto a stable support to assist balance for items 23-25)
				/2	23. ABDUCTS AFFECTED HIP WITH KNEE EXTENDED *"Keep your knee straight and your hips level, and raise your leg to the side"*
				/2	24. FLEXES AFFECTED KNEE WITH HIP EXTENDED *"Keep your hip straight, bend your knee back and bring your heel towards your bottom"*
				/2	25. DORSIFLEXES AFFECTED ANKLE WITH KNEE EXTENDED *"Keep your heel on the ground and lift your toes off the floor as far as you can"* Note: affected foot is placed slightly forward in position of a small step (heel in line with toes of other foot).
					STANDING AND WALKING ACTIVITIES
				/3	26. PLACES AFFECTED FOOT ONTO FIRST STEP (or stool 18-cm high) *"Lift your foot and place it onto the first step (or stool) in front of you"* Note: returning the foot to the ground is not scored; use of handrail =aid (score 2).
				/3	27. TAKES 3 STEPS BACKWARDS (one and a half gait cycles) *"Take three average sized steps backwards, placing one foot behind the other"*
				/3	28. TAKES 3 STEPS SIDEWAYS TO AFFECTED SIDE *"Take three average sized steps sideways towards your weak side"*
				/3	29. WALKS 10 METERS INDOORS (on smooth, obstacle-free surface) *"Walk in a straight line over to ... (a specified point 10 meters away)"* Note: orthotic=aid (score 2); longer than 20 seconds =marked deviation (score 1c).
				/3	30. WALKS DOWN 3 STAIRS ALTERNATING FEET *"Walk down three stairs; place only one foot at a time on each step if you can"* Note: handrail=aid (score 2); non-alternating feet=marked deviation (score 1a or 1c).

*The STREAM scoring form and criteria are presented verbatim. CVA=cerebrovascular accident, ROM=range of motion.

1. Daley K, Mayo NE, Wood-Dauphinée SL, et al. Verification of the Stroke Rehabilitation Assessment of Movement (STREAM). Physiotherapy Canada.1997;49:269-78.
2. Daley K, Mayo NE, Wood-Dauphinée SL. Reliability of scores on the Stroke Rehabilitation Assessment of Movement (STREAM) measure. Phys Ther.1999;79:8-19.
3. Ahmed S, Mayo NE, Higgins J, Salbach NM, Finch L, Wood-Dauphinée S L. The Stroke Rehabilitation Assessment of Movement (STREAM): A Comparison With Other Measures Used to Evaluate Effects of Stroke and Rehabilitation, Physical Therapy. July 2003:83(7);617-30

Appendix VI

Unified Parkinson's Disease Rating Scale (UPDRS)

I. MENTATION, BEHAVIOR AND MOOD

1. **Intellectual Impairment**
   - 0 = None.
   - 1 = Mild. Consistent forgetfulness with partial recollection of events and no other difficulties.
   - 2 = Moderate memory loss, with disorientation and moderate difficulty handling complex problems.
   - Mild but definite impairment of function at home with need of occasional prompting.
   - 3 = Severe memory loss with disorientation for time and often to place.
   - Severe impairment in handling problems.
   - 4 = Severe memory loss with orientation preserved to person only. Unable to make judgements or solve problems. Requires much help with personal care. Cannot be left alone at all.
2. **Thought Disorder** (Due to dementia or drug intoxication)
   - 0 = None.
   - 1 = Vivid dreaming.
   - 2 = "Benign" hallucinations with insight retained.
   - 3 = Occasional to frequent hallucinations or delusions; without insight; could interfere with daily activities.
   - 4 = Persistent hallucinations, delusions, or florrid psychosis. Not able to care for self.
3. **Depression**
   - 0 = None.
   - 1 = Periods of sadness or guilt greater than normal, never sustained for days or weeks.
   - 2 = Sustained depression (1 week or more).

- 3 = Sustained depression with vegetative symptoms (insomnia, anorexia, weight loss, loss of interest).
- 4 = Sustained depression with vegetative symptoms and suicidal thoughts or intent.

4. **Motivation/Initiative**
    - 0 = Normal.
    - 1 = Less assertive than usual; more passive.
    - 2 = Loss of initiative or disinterest in elective (nonroutine) activities.
    - 3 = Loss of initiative or disinterest in day-to-day (routine) activities.
    - 4 = Withdrawn, complete loss of motivation.

II. ACTIVITIES OF DAILY LIVING (FOR BOTH "ON" AND "OFF")

5. **Speech**
    - 0 = Normal.
    - 1 = Mildly affected. No difficulty being understood.
    - 2 = Moderately affected. Sometimes asked to repeat statements.
    - 3 = Severely affected. Frequently asked to repeat statements.
    - 4 = Unintelligible most of the time.
6. **Salivation**
    - 0 = Normal.
    - 1 = Slight but definite excess of saliva in mouth; may have nighttime drooling.
    - 2 = Moderately excessive saliva; may have minimal drooling.
    - 3 = Marked excess of saliva with some drooling.
    - 4 = Marked drooling, requires constant tissue or handkerchief.
7. **Swallowing**
    - 0 = Normal.
    - 1 = Rare choking.
    - 2 = Occasional choking.
    - 3 = Requires soft food.
    - 4 = Requires NG tube or gastrotomy feeding.
8. **Handwriting**
    - 0 = Normal.
    - 1 = Slightly slow or small.
    - 2 = Moderately slow or small; all words are legible.
    - 3 = Severely affected; not all words are legible.
    - 4 = The majority of words are not legible.

9. **Cutting food and handling utensils**
    - 0 = Normal.
    - 1 = Somewhat slow and clumsy, but no help needed.
    - 2 = Can cut most foods, although clumsy and slow; some help needed.
    - 3 = Food must be cut by someone, but can still feed slowly.
    - 4 = Needs to be fed.
10. **Dressing**
    - 0 = Normal.
    - 1 = Somewhat slow, but no help needed.
    - 2 = Occasional assistance with buttoning, getting arms in sleeves.
    - 3 = Considerable help required, but can do some things alone.
    - 4 = Helpless.
11. **Hygiene**
    - 0 = Normal.
    - 1 = Somewhat slow, but no help needed.
    - 2 = Needs help to shower or bathe; or very slow in hygienic care.
    - 3 = Requires assistance for washing, brushing teeth, combing hair, going to bathroom.
    - 4 = Foley catheter or other mechanical aids.
12. **Turning in bed and adjusting bed clothes**
    - 0 = Normal.
    - 1 = Somewhat slow and clumsy, but no help needed.
    - 2 = Can turn alone or adjust sheets, but with great difficulty.
    - 3 = Can initiate, but not turn or adjust sheets alone.
    - 4 = Helpless.
13. **Falling** (unrelated to freezing)
    - 0 = None.
    - 1 = Rare falling.
    - 2 = Occasionally falls, less than once per day.
    - 3 = Falls an average of once daily.
    - 4 = Falls more than once daily.
14. **Freezing when walking**
    - 0 = None.
    - 1 = Rare freezing when walking; may have starthesitation.
    - 2 = Occasional freezing when walking.
    - 3 = Frequent freezing. Occasionally falls from freezing.
    - 4 = Frequent falls from freezing.

15. **Walking**
    - 0 = Normal.
    - 1 = Mild difficulty. May not swing arms or may tend to drag leg.
    - 2 = Moderate difficulty, but requires little or no assistance.
    - 3 = Severe disturbance of walking, requiring assistance.
    - 4 = Cannot walk at all, even with assistance.
16. **Tremor** (Symptomatic complaint of tremor in any part of body)
    - 0 = Absent.
    - 1 = Slight and infrequently present.
    - 2 = Moderate; bothersome to patient.
    - 3 = Severe; interferes with many activities.
    - 4 = Marked; interferes with most activities.
17. **Sensory complaints related to parkinsonism**
    - 0 = None.
    - 1 = Occasionally has numbness, tingling, or mild aching.
    - 2 = Frequently has numbness, tingling, or aching; not distressing.
    - 3 = Frequent painful sensations.
    - 4 = Excruciating pain.

III. MOTOR EXAMINATION

18. **Speech**
    - 0 = Normal.
    - 1 = Slight loss of expression, diction and/or volume.
    - 2 = Monotone, slurred but understandable; moderately impaired.
    - 3 = Marked impairment, difficult to understand.
    - 4 = Unintelligible.
19. **Facial expression**
    - 0 = Normal.
    - 1 = Minimal hypomimia, could be normal "Poker Face".
    - 2 = Slight but definitely abnormal diminution of facial expression.
    - 3 = Moderate hypomimia; lips parted some of the time.
    - 4 = Masked or fixed facies with severe or complete loss of facial expression; lips parted 1/4 inch or more.
20. **Tremor at rest** (head, upper and lower extremities)
    - 0 = Absent.

- 1 = Slight and infrequently present.
- 2 = Mild in amplitude and persistent. Or moderate in amplitude, but only intermittently present.
- 3 = Moderate in amplitude and present most of the time.
- 4 = Marked in amplitude and present most of the time.

21. **Action or postural tremor of hands**
    - 0 = Absent.
    - 1 = Slight; present with action.
    - 2 = Moderate in amplitude, present with action.
    - 3 = Moderate in amplitude with posture holding as well as action.
    - 4 = Marked in amplitude; interferes with feeding.
22. **Rigidity** (judged on passive movement of major joints with patient relaxed in sitting position.
    - Cogwheeling to be ignored.)
    - 0 = Absent.
    - 1 = Slight or detectable only when activated by mirror or other movements.
    - 2 = Mild to moderate.
    - 3 = Marked, but full range of motion easily achieved.
    - 4 = Severe, range of motion achieved with difficulty.
23. **Finger taps** (patient taps thumb with index finger in rapid succession.)
    - 0 = Normal.
    - 1 = Mild slowing and/or reduction in amplitude.
    - 2 = Moderately impaired. Definite and early fatiguing. May have occasional arrests in movement.
    - 3 = Severely impaired. Frequent hesitation in initiating movements or arrests in ongoing movement.
    - 4 = Can barely perform the task.
24. **Hand movements** (patient opens and closes hands in rapid succesion)
    - 0 = Normal.
    - 1 = Mild slowing and/or reduction in amplitude.
    - 2 = Moderately impaired. Definite and early fatiguing. May have occasional arrests in movement.
    - 3 = Severely impaired. Frequent hesitation in initiating movements or arrests in ongoing movement.
    - 4 = Can barely perform the task.

25. **Rapid alternating movements of hands** (pronation-supination movements of hands, vertically and horizontally, with as large an amplitude as possible, both hands simultaneously.)
    - 0 = Normal.
    - 1 = Mild slowing and/or reduction in amplitude.
    - 2 = Moderately impaired. Definite and early fatiguing. May have occasional arrests in movement.
    - 3 = Severely impaired. Frequent hesitation in initiating movements or arrests in ongoing movement.
    - 4 = Can barely perform the task.
26. **Leg agility** (Patient taps heel on the ground in rapid succession picking up entire leg. Amplitude should be at least 3 inches.)
    - 0 = Normal.
    - 1 = Mild slowing and/or reduction in amplitude.
    - 2 = Moderately impaired. Definite and early fatiguing. May have occasional arrests in movement.
    - 3 = Severely impaired. Frequent hesitation in initiating movements or arrests in ongoing movement.
    - 4 = Can barely perform the task.
27. **Arising from chair**

    (Patient attempts to rise from a straightbacked chair, with arms folded across chest)
    - 0 = Normal.
    - 1 = Slow; or may need more than one attempt.
    - 2 = Pushes self up from arms of seat.
    - 3 = Tends to fall back and may have to try more than one time, but can get up without help.
    - 4 = Unable to arise without help.
28. **Posture**
    - 0 = Normal erect.
    - 1 = Not quite erect, slightly stooped posture; could be normal for older person.
    - 2 = Moderately stooped posture, definitely abnormal; can be slightly leaning to one side.
    - 3 = Severely stooped posture with kyphosis; can be moderately leaning to one side.
    - 4 = Marked flexion with extreme abnormality of posture.
29. **Gait**
    - 0 = Normal.
    - 1 = Walks slowly, may shuffle with short steps, but no festination (hastening steps) or propulsion.

- 2 = Walks with difficulty, but requires little or no assistance; may have some festination, short steps, or propulsion.
- 3 = Severe disturbance of gait, requiring assistance.
- 4 = Cannot walk at all, even with assistance.

30. **Postural stability** (response to sudden, strong posterior displacement produced by pull on shoulders while patient erect with eyes open and feet slightly apart. Patient is prepared.)
    - 0 = Normal.
    - 1 = Retropulsion, but recovers unaided.
    - 2 = Absence of postural response; would fall if not caught by examiner.
    - 3 = Very unstable, tends to lose balance spontaneously.
    - 4 = Unable to stand without assistance.
31. **Body bradykinesia and hypokinesia** (combining slowness, hesitancy, decreased armswing, small amplitude and poverty of movement in general)
    - 0 = None.
    - 1 = Minimal slowness, giving movement a deliberate character; could be normal for some persons. Possibly reduced amplitude.
    - 2 = Mild degree of slowness and poverty of movement which is definitely abnormal. Alternatively, some reduced amplitude.
    - 3 = Moderate slowness, poverty or small amplitude of movement.
    - 4 = Marked slowness, poverty or small amplitude of movement.

IV. COMPLICATIONS OF THERAPY (In the Past Week)

A. Dyskinesias

32. **Duration: What proportion of the waking day are dyskinesias present?**
    (Historical information)
    - 0 = None
    - 1 = 1–25% of day.
    - 2 = 26–50% of day.
    - 3 = 51–75% of day.
    - 4 = 76–100% of day.

33. **Disability: How disabling are the dyskinesias?**
(Historical information; may be modified by office examination)
    - 0 = Not disabling.
    - 1 = Mildly disabling.
    - 2 = Moderately disabling.
    - 3 = Severely disabling.
    - 4 = Completely disabled.
34. **Painful dyskinesias: How painful are the dyskinesias?**
    - 0 = No painful dyskinesias.
    - 1 = Slight.
    - 2 = Moderate.
    - 3 = Severe.
    - 4 = Marked.
35. **Presence of early morning dystonia** (Historical information.)
    - 0 = No
    - 1 = Yes

B. Clinical Fluctuations

36. **Are "off" periods predictable?**
    - 0 = No
    - 1 = Yes
37. **Are "off" periods unpredictable?**
    - 0 = No
    - 1 = Yes
38. **Do "off" periods come on suddenly, within a few seconds?**
    - 0 = No
    - 1 = Yes
39. **What proportion of the waking day is the patient "off" on average?**
    - 0 = None
    - 1 = 1–25% of day.
    - 2 = 26–50% of day.
    - 3 = 51–75% of day.
    - 4 = 76–100% of day.

C. Other Complications

40. **Does the patient have anorexia, nausea, or vomiting?**
    - 0 = No
    - 1 = Yes

41. **Any sleep disturbances, such as insomnia or hypersomnolence?**
    - 0 = No
    - 1 = Yes
42. **Does the patient have symptomatic orthostasis?**
    (Record the patient's blood pressure, height and weight on the scoring form)
    - 0 = No
    - 1 = Yes

V. MODIFIED HOEHN AND YAHR STAGING

- Stage 0 = No signs of disease.
- Stage 1 = Unilateral disease.
- Stage 1.5 = Unilateral plus axial involvement.
- Stage 2 = Bilateral disease, without impairment of balance.
- Stage 2.5 = Mild bilateral disease, with recovery on pull test.
- Stage 3 = Mild to moderate bilateral disease; some postural instability; physically independent.
- Stage 4 = Severe disability; still able to walk or stand unassisted.
- Stage 5 = Wheelchair bound or bedridden unless aided.

VI. SCHWAB AND ENGLAND ACTIVITIES OF DAILY LIVING SCALE

- 100% = Completely independent. Able to do all chores without slowness, difficulty or impairment.
- Essentially normal. Unaware of any difficulty.
- 90% = Completely independent. Able to do all chores with some degree of slowness, difficulty and impairment. Might take twice as long. Beginning to be aware of difficulty.
- 80% = Completely independent in most chores. Takes twice as long. Conscious of difficulty and slowness.
- 70% = Not completely independent. More difficulty with some chores. Three to four times as long in some. Must spend a large part of the day with chores.
- 60% = Some dependency. Can do most chores, but exceedingly slowly and with much effort. Errors; some impossible.
- 50% = More dependent. Help with half, slower, etc. Difficulty with everything.

- 40% = Very dependent. Can assist with all chores, but few alone.
- 30% = With effort, now and then does a few chores alone or begins alone. Much help needed.
- 20% = Nothing alone. Can be a slight help with some chores. Severe invalid.
- 10% = Totally dependent, helpless. Complete invalid.
- 0% = Vegetative functions such as swallowing, bladder and bowel functions are not functioning. Bedridden.

BIBLIOGRAPHY

1. Canter CJ, de la Torre R, Mier M. A method of evaluating disability in patients with Parkinson's disease. J Nerv Ment Dis 1961;133:143-7.
2. Louis ED, Lynch T, Marder K, et al. Reliability of patient completion of the historical section of the Unified Parkinson's disease Rating Scale. Mov Disord. 1996;11:185-92.
3. Van Hilten JJ, van der Zwan AD, Zwinderman AH, et al. Rating impairment and disability in Parkinson's disease: evaluation of the Unified Parkinson's disease Rating Scale. Mov Disord. 1994;9:84-8.

Appendix VII

The Trunk Control Test for Motor Impairment After Stroke

OVERVIEW

The Trunk Control Test can be used to assess the motor impairment in a patient who has had a stroke. It correlates with eventual walking ability. Testing done by patient lying on bed:

1. Roll to weak side
2. Roll to strong side
3. Balance in sitting position on the edge of the bed with the feet off the ground for at least 30 seconds
4. Sit up from lying down

Scoring Each Test	Points
▪ Unable to do without assistance	0
▪ Able to do so using nonmuscular help or in an abnormal style;	12
▪ Uses arms to steady self when sitting able to complete task normally	25
▪ Trunk control test = SUM (points for all 4 tests)	

Interpretation

- Minimum score: 0
- Maximum score: 100
- If the test is done at 6 weeks after stroke a score >= 50 predicts recovery of the ability to walk by 18 weeks.

BIBLIOGRAPHY

1. Franchignoni FP, Tesio L, Ricupero C, Martino MT, Trunk Control Test as an Early Predictor of Stroke Rehabilitation Outcome Stroke.1997; 28: 1382-5
2. Collin C Wade D. Assessing motor impairment after stroke: a pilot reliability study. J Neurology Neurosurg. Psychiatry. 1990;53:576-9

Appendix VIII

Dynamic Gait Index

Patient: ______________________________________ Date: ___________

1. Gait level surface _____

Instructions: Walk at your normal speed from here to the next mark (20')

Grading: Mark the lowest category that applies:

Normal (3)**:** Walks 20′, no assistive devices, good speed, no evidence for imbalance, normal gait pattern.
Mild Impairment (2): Walks 20′, uses assistive devices, slower speed, mild gait deviations.
Moderate Impairment (1): Walks 20′, slow speed, abnormal gait pattern, ev idence for imbalance.
Severe Impairment (0): Cannot walk 20′ without assistance, severe gait deviations or imbalance.

2. Change in gait speed _____

Instructions: Begin walking at your normal pace (for 5′), when I tell you "go," walk as fast as you can (for 5′). When I tell you "slow," walk as slowly as you can (for 5′).

Grading: Mark the lowest category that applies.

Normal (3): Able to smoothly change walking speed without loss of balance or gait deviation. Shows a significant difference in walking speeds between normal, fast and slow speeds.
Mild impairment (2): Is able to change speed but demonstrates mild gait deviations, or no gait deviations but is unable to achieve a significant change in velocity, or uses an assistive device.
Moderate impairment (1): Makes only minor adjustments to walking speed, or accomplishes a change in speed with significant gait deviations, or changes speed but loses significant gait deviations, or changes speed but loses balance but is able to recover and continue walking.

Severe impairment (0): Cannot change speeds, or loses balance and has to reach for wall or be caught.

3. Gait with horizontal head turns _____

Instructions: Begin walking at your normal pace. When I tell you to "look right," keep walking straight, but turn your head to the right. Keep looking to the right until I tell you, "look left," then keep walking straight and turn your head to the left. Keep your head to the left until I tell you "look straight," then keep walking straight, but return your head to the center.

Grading: Mark the lowest category that applies.

Normal (3): Performs head turns smoothly with no change in gait.
Mild impairment (2): Performs head turns smoothly with slight change in gait velocity, i.e. minor disruption to smooth gait path or uses walking aid.
Moderate impairment (1): Performs head turns with moderate change in gait velocity, slows down, staggers but recovers, can continue to walk.
Severe impairment (0): Performs task with severe disruption of gait, i.e., staggers, outside 15" path, loses balance, stops, reac hes for wall.

4. Gait with vertical head turns _____

Instructions: Begin walking at your normal pace. When I tell you to "look up," keep walking straight, but tip your head up. Keep looking up until I tell you, "look down," then keep walking straight and tip your head down. Keep your head down until I tell you "look straight," then keep walking straight, but return your head to the center.

Grading: Mark the lowest category that applies.

Normal (3): Performs head turns smoothly with no change in gait.
Mild impairment (2): Performs task with slight change in gait velocity, i.e., minor disruption to smooth gait path or uses walking aid.
Moderate impairment (1): Performs task with moderate change in gait velocity, slows down, staggers but recovers, can continue to walk.
Severe impairment (0): Performs task with severe disruption of gait, i.e., staggers, outside 15″ path, loses balance, stops, reaches for wall.

5. Gait and pivot turn _____

Instructions: Begin walking at your normal pace. When I tell you, "turn and stop," turn as quickly as you can to face the opposite direction and stop.

Grading: Mark the lowest category that applies.

Normal (3): Pivot turns safely within 3 seconds and stops quickly with no loss of balance.
Mild impairment (2): Pivot turns safely in > 3 seconds and stops with no loss of balance.
Moderate Impairment (1): Turns slowly, requires verbal cueing, requires several small steps to catch balance following turn and stop.
Severe Impairment (0): Cannot turn safely, requires assistance to turn and stop.

6. Step over obstacle ____

Instructions: Begin walking at your normal speed. When you come to the shoebox, step over it, not around it, and keep walking.
Grading: Mark the lowest category that applies.
Normal (3): Is able to step over the box without changing gait speed, no evidence of imbalance.
Mild impairment (2): Is able to step ov er box, but must slow down and adjust steps to clear box safely.
Moderate impairment (1): Is able to step over box but must stop, then step over. May require verbal cueing.
Severe impairment (0): Cannot perform without assistance.

7. Step around obstacles _____

Instructions: Begin walking at normal speed. When you come to the firs t cone (about 6′ away), walk around the right side of it. When you come to the second cone (6′ past first cone), walk around it to the left.

Grading: Mark the lowest category that applies.

Normal (3): Is able to walk around cones safely without changing gait speed; no evidence of imbalance.
Mild impairment (2): Is able to step around both cones, but must slow down and adjust steps to clear cones .
Moderate impairment (1): Is able to clear cones but must significantly slow speed to accomplish task, or requires verbal cueing.
Severe impairment (0): Unable to clear cones, walks into one or both cones, or requires physical assistance.

8. Steps _____

Instructions: Walk up these stairs as you would at home, i.e. using the railing if necessary. At the top, turn around and walk down.

Grading: Mark the lowest category that applies.

Normal (3): Alternating feet, no rail.
Mild impairment (2): Alternating feet, must use rail.
Moderate impairment (1): Two feet to a stair, must use rail.
Severe impairment (0): Cannot do safely.
Total Score: ___ / 24
Scoring Informatio n: 21/24 or above = minimal to no risk for falls
Below 21 indicates risk for falls and the lower the score, the more the risk

BIBLIOGRAPHY

1. Common score for moderate sta ge Parkinson Disease = 9 -11/24.
2. Herman T, Inbar-Borovsky N, Brozgol M, Giladi N, Hausdorff JM. The Dynamic Gait index in healthy older adults: the role of stair climbing, fear of falling and gender. Gait Posture. 2009 Feb;29(2):237-41.
3. Jonsdottir J, Cattaneo D. Reliability and validity of the dynamic gait index in persons with chronic stroke. Arch Phys Med Rehabil. 2007 Nov; 88(11):1410–5.
4. Lin JH, Hsu MJ, Hsu HW, Wu HC, Hsieh CL. Psychometric Comparisons of 3 functional ambulation measures for patients with stroke. Stroke. 2010

Appendix IX

Berg Balance Scale

BERG BALANCE SCALE

The berg balance scale (BBS) was developed to measure balance among older people with impairment in balance function by assessing the performance of functional tasks. It is a valid instrument used for evaluation of the effectiveness of interventions and for quantitative descriptions of function in clinical practice and research. The BBS has been evaluated in several reliability studies. A recent study of the BBS, which was completed in Finland, indicates that a change of eight (8) BBS points is required to reveal a genuine change in function between two assessments among older people who are dependent in ADL and living in residential care facilities.

Description:

- 14-item scale designed to measure balance of the older adult in a clinical setting.
- Equipment needed: Ruler, two standard chairs (one with arm rests, one without), footstool or step, stopwatch or wristwatch, 15 feet walkway
- Completion: Time: 15–20 minutes
- Scoring: A five-point scale, ranging from 0–4. "0" indicates the lowest level of function and "4" the highest level of function. Total score = 56
- Interpretation: 41–56 = low fall risk
- 21–40 = medium fall risk
- 0–20 = high fall risk
- A change of 8 points is required to reveal a genuine change in function between 2 assessments.

Name: ________________________________ Date: __________
Location: ______________________________ Rater: __________
Item description score (0–4)
Sitting to standing ________
Standing unsupported ________
Sitting unsupported ________
Standing to sitting ________
Transfers ________
Standing with eyes closed ________
Standing with feet together ________
Reaching forward with outstretched arm ________
Retrieving object from floor ________
Turning to look behind ________
Turning 360 degrees ________
Placing alternate foot on stool ________
Standing with one foot in front ________
Standing on one foot ________
Total ________

General Instructions

Please document each task and/or give instructions as written. When scoring, please record the lowest response category that applies for each item.

In most items, the subject is asked to maintain a given position for a specific time. Progressively more points are deducted if:

- The time or distance requirements are not met
- The subject's performance warrants supervision
- The subject touches an external support or receives assistance from the examiner.

Subject should understand that they must maintain their balance while attempting the tasks. The choices of which leg to stand on or how far to reach are left to the subject. Poor judgment will adversely influence the performance and the scoring.

Equipment required for testing is a stopwatch or watch with a second hand, and a ruler or other indicator of 2, 5, and 10 inches. Chairs used during testing should be a reasonable height. Either a step or a stool of average step height may be used for item # 12.

SITTING TO STANDING

Instructions: Please stand up. Try not to use your hand for support.
( ) 4 able to stand without using hands and stabilize independently
( ) 3 able to stand independently using hands
( ) 2 able to stand using hands after several tries
( ) 1 needs minimal aid to stand or stabilize
( ) 0 needs moderate or maximal assist to stand

STANDING UNSUPPORTED

Instructions: Please stand for 2 minutes without holding on.
( ) 4 able to stand safely for 2 minutes
( ) 3 able to stand 2 minutes with supervision
( ) 2 able to stand 30 seconds unsupported
( ) 1 needs several tries to stand 30 seconds unsupported
( ) 0 unable to stand 30 seconds unsupported
If a subject is able to stand 2 minutes unsupported, score full points for sitting unsupported. Proceed to item #4.

SITTING WITH BACK UNSUPPORTED BUT FEET SUPPORTED ON FLOOR OR ON A STOOL

Instructions: Please sit with arms folded for 2 minutes.
( ) 4 able to sit safely and securely for 2 minutes
( ) 3 able to sit 2 minutes under supervision
( ) 2 able to ableto sit 30 seconds
( ) 1 able to sit 10 seconds
( ) 0 unable to sit without support 10 seconds

STANDING TO SITTING

Instructions: Please sit down.
( ) 4 sits safely with minimal use of hands
( ) 3 controls descent by using hands
( ) 2 uses back of legs against chair to control descent
( ) 1 sits independently but has uncontrolled descent
( ) 0 needs assist to sit

Transfers

Instructions: Arrange chair(s) for pivot transfer. Ask subject to transfer one way toward a seat with armrests and one way toward a seat without armrests. You may use two chairs (one with and one without armrests) or a bed and a chair.
( ) 4 able to transfer safely with minor use of hands
( ) 3 able to transfer safely definite need of hands
( ) 2 able to transfer with verbal cuing and/or supervision
( ) 1 needs one person to assist
( ) 0 needs two people to assist or supervise to be safe.

Standing Unsupported with Eyes Closed

Instructions: Please close your eyes and stand still for 10 seconds.
( ) 4 able to stand 10 seconds safely
( ) 3 able to stand 10 seconds with supervision
( ) 2 able to stand 3 seconds
( ) 1 unable to keep eyes closed 3 seconds but stays safely
( ) 0 needs help to keep from falling.

Standing Unsupported with Feet Together

Instructions: Place your feet together and stand without holding on.
( ) 4 able to place feet together independently and stand 1 minute safely
( ) 3 able to place feet together independently and stand 1 minute with supervision
( ) 2 able to place feet together independently but unable to hold for 30 seconds
( ) 1 needs help to attain position but able to stand 15 seconds feet together
( ) 0 needs help to attain position and unable to hold for 15 seconds.

Reaching Forward with Outstretched arm While Standing

Instructions: Lift arm to 90°. Stretch out your fingers and reach forward as far as you can. (Examiner places a ruler at the end of fingertips when arm is at 90°. Fingers should not touch the ruler while reaching forward. The recorded measure is the distance forward that the fingers reach while the subject is in the most forward lean position. When possible, ask subject to use both arms when reaching to avoid rotation of the trunk.)

( ) 4 can reach forward confidently 25 cm (10 inches)
( ) 3 can reach forward 12 cm (5 inches)
( ) 2 can reach forward 5 cm (2 inches)
( ) 1 reaches forward but needs supervision
( ) 0 loses balance while trying/requires external support.

Pick up Object from the Floor from a Standing Position

Instructions: Pick up the shoe/slipper, which is in front of your feet.
( ) 4 able to pick up slipper safely and easily
( ) 3 able to pick up slipper but needs supervision
( ) 2 unable to pick up but reaches 2–5 cm (1–2 inches) from slipper and keeps balance independently
( ) 1 unable to pick up and needs supervision while trying
( ) 0 unable to try/needs assist to keep from losing balance or falling.

Turning to Look Behind Over Left and Right Shoulders While Standing

Instructions: Turn to look directly behind you over toward the left shoulder. Repeat to the right. (Examiner may pick an object to look at directly behind the subject to encourage a better twist turn.)
( ) 4 looks behind from both sides and weight shifts well
( ) 3 looks behind one side only other side shows less weight shift
( ) 2 turns sideways only but maintains balance
( ) 1 needs supervision when turning
( ) 0 needs assist to keep from losing balance or falling.

Turn 360°

Instructions: Turn completely around in a full circle. Pause. Then turn a full circle in the other direction.
( ) 4 able to turn 360° safely in 4 seconds or less
( ) 3 able to turn 360° safely one side only 4 seconds or less
( ) 2 able to turn 360° safely but slowly
( ) 1 needs close supervision or verbal cuing
( ) 0 needs assistance while turning.

Place Alternate Foot on Step or Stool While Standing Unsupported

Instructions: Place each foot alternately on the step/stool. Continue until each foot has touched the step/stool four times.

( ) 4 able to stand independently and safely and complete 8 steps in 20 seconds
( ) 3 able to stand independently and complete 8 steps in > 20 seconds
( ) 2 able to complete 4 steps without aid with supervision
( ) 1 able to complete > 2 steps needs minimal assist
( ) 0 needs assistance to keep from falling/unable to try

Standing Unsupported one Foot in Front

Instructions (Demonstrate to Subject): Place one foot directly in front of the other. If you feel that you cannot place your foot directly in front, try to step far enough ahead that the heel of your forward foot is ahead of the toes of the other foot. (To score 3 points, the length of the step should exceed the length of the other foot and the width of the stance should approximate the subject's normal stride width.)

( ) 4 able to place foot tandem independently and hold 30 seconds
( ) 3 able to place foot ahead independently and hold 30 seconds
( ) 2 able to take small step independently and hold 30 seconds
( ) 1 needs help to step but can hold 15 seconds
( ) 0 loses balance while stepping or standing

Standing on One Leg

Instructions: Stand on one leg as long as you can without holding on.

( ) 4 able to lift leg independently and hold >10 seconds
( ) 3 able to lift leg independently and hold 5–10 seconds
( ) 2 able to lift leg independently and hold = 3 seconds
( ) 1 tries to lift leg unable to hold 3 seconds but remains standing independently.
( ) 0 unable to try of needs assist to prevent fall
( ) Total Score (Maximum = 56)

BIBLIOGRAPHY

1. Berg K, Wood-Dauphinee S, Williams JI, Gayton D. Measuring balance in the elderly: Preliminary development of an instrument. Physiotherapy Canada, 41:304–11, 1989.
2. Berg K, Wood-Dauphinee S, Williams JI, Maki, B. Measuring balance in the elderly: Validation of an instrument. Can. J. Pub. Health, July/August supplement, 2:S7–11, 1992.
3. Berg K, et al (1995). The balance scale: reliability assessment for elderly residents and patients with an acute stroke. Scandinavian Journal of Rehabilitation Medicine, 27, 27–36.

Index

D

E

F

K

L

M

N

O

P

Q

R

S